Patient Care Guidelines
for Nurse Practitioners

Patient Care Guidelines for Nurse Practitioners
Third Edition

Edited by

Axalla J. Hoole, M.D.
Associate Professor of Medicine,
University of North Carolina at Chapel Hill
School of Medicine; Associate Attending
Physician, Department of Medicine,
North Carolina Memorial Hospital,
Chapel Hill, North Carolina

Robert A. Greenberg, M.D.
Professor of Pediatrics, University of
North Carolina at Chapel Hill School of
Medicine; Attending Physician,
Department of Pediatrics, North Carolina
Memorial Hospital, Chapel Hill, North
Carolina

C. Glenn Pickard, Jr., M.D.
Professor of Medicine, University of
North Carolina at Chapel Hill School of
Medicine; Attending Physician,
Department of Medicine, North Carolina
Memorial Hospital, Chapel Hill, North
Carolina

Little, Brown and Company
Boston   Toronto

Library of Congress Cataloging-in-Publication Data

Patient care guidelines for nurse practitioners.

Includes index.
1. Nurse practitioners. 2. Medical protocols.
I. Hoole, Axalla J., 1938–   . II. Greenberg,
Robert A. (Robert Aaron), 1938–   . III. Pickard,
C. Glenn (Carl Glenn), 1936–   . [DNLM: 1. Nurse
Practitioners—handbooks. 2. Nursing—handbooks.
WY 39 P298]
RT82.8.P37   1987   616′.0024613   87–3785
ISBN 0–316–37230–7

Library of Congress Catalog Card No. 87–3785

ISBN 0-673-39376-3

9 8 7 6 5 4 3

SEM

Printed in the United States of America

Contents

Contributing Authors

Timothy S. Carey, M.D.   Assistant Professor of Medicine, University of North Carolina at Chapel Hill School of Medicine; Assistant Attending Physician, Department of Medicine, North Carolina Memorial Hospital, Chapel Hill, North Carolina

Lamar E. Ekbladh, M.D.   Associate Professor, Milton S. Hershey Medical Center, Department of Obstetrics and Gynecology, Hershey, Pennsylvania

Robert A. Greenberg, M.D.   Professor of Pediatrics, University of North Carolina at Chapel Hill School of Medicine; Attending Physician, Department of Pediatrics, North Carolina Memorial Hospital, Chapel Hill, North Carolina

Sandra Hak, Pharm. D.   Clinical Assistant Professor of Pharmacy, University of North Carolina School of Pharmacy

Harvey J. Hamrick, M.D.   Associate Professor of Pediatrics, University of North Carolina at Chapel Hill School of Medicine; Attending Physician and Director of the Pediatric Primary Care Clinic, Department of Pediatrics, North Carolina Memorial Hospital, Chapel Hill, North Carolina

Axalla J. Hoole, M.D.   Associate Professor of Medicine, University of North Carolina at Chapel Hill School of Medicine; Associate Attending Physician, Department of Medicine, North Carolina Memorial Hospital, Chapel Hill, North Carolina

Robert S. Lawrence, M.D.   Associate Professor of Medicine and Director, Division of Primary Care, Harvard Medical School, Boston; Director of Medicine, The Cambridge Hospital, Cambridge, Massachusetts

Gregory S. Liptak,
M.D., M.P.H.

George Washington Goler Associate Professor of Pediatrics, University of Rochester School of Medicine and Dentistry; Director of Birth Defects Center, Department of Pediatrics, Strong Memorial Hospital, Rochester, New York

Frank A. Loda, M.D.

Professor of Pediatrics and Adjunct Professor of Maternal and Child Health, University of North Carolina at Chapel Hill School of Medicine; Attending Physician and Division Chief of Community Pediatrics, Department of Pediatrics, North Carolina Memorial Hospital, Chapel Hill, North Carolina

C. Glenn Pickard, Jr., M.D.

Professor of Medicine, University of North Carolina at Chapel Hill School of Medicine; Attending Physician, Department of Medicine, North Carolina Memorial Hospital, Chapel Hill, North Carolina

Samuel M. Putnam, M.D.

Associate Professor of Medicine and Director of Medical Residency Program, Saint Mary's Hospital, Rochester, New York

James E. Schwankl,
M.D., M.P.H.

Clinical Assistant Professor of Pediatrics, University of North Carolina at Chapel Hill School of Medicine; Attending Physician, Chatham Hospital, Siler City, North Carolina

Edward H. Wagner,
M.D., M.P.H.

Professor of Health Services, University of Washington School of Public Health and Community Medicine, Department of Health Services; Director, Center for Health Studies, Group Health Cooperative of Puget Sound, Seattle, Washington

Nelson A. Warner, M.D.

Attending Dermatologist and Vice Chairman, Medical Education, Winter Haven Hospital, Winter Haven, Florida

Preface

In the decade from 1965 to 1975, the United States was confronted with a medical care "crisis" involving the quality, quantity, and accessibility of primary health care services that particularly affected the rural areas and the inner cities. The disappearance of the general practitioner from small towns and villages in rural areas and the flight of physicians from the inner cities to the suburbs created major problems in medical care delivery that stimulated a wide variety of programs designed to alleviate the crisis.

As one response to this crisis, the Schools of Nursing, Public Health, and Medicine at the University of North Carolina at Chapel Hill developed a training program for Family Nurse Practitioners (FNPs). In conjunction with the training program, faculty members of the schools participated in an innovative primary health care delivery program in which FNPs staffed satellite rural clinics while physicians from the medical center provided consultation and supervision for the medical practice of the FNPs.

The patient care guidelines presented in this manual were initially developed in the training program and the demonstration practice. Subsequently, they have been modified and changed repeatedly based on our own experience and the experience of others across the nation who are engaged in similar practices. They still represent our approach to management. Accordingly, this book is not intended as an exhaustive treatise on the conditions covered nor as an exposition of all the ways in which each condition can be managed. Rather, it is intended as a code of acceptable criteria for diagnosing an illness or condition and of acceptable plans for management.

Although many individuals are predicting that as more physicians are trained and enter practice, the importance of the nurse practitioner will decline, we have found, rather, a shift in locations. Many nurse practitioners are still in practice in rural satellite clinics, but in recent years an increasing number have gone to large urban clinics, particularly to HMOs, to highly specialized areas of practice such as oncology clinics, and to rest and retirement homes, where nurse practitioners often assume the role of the primary coordinator of care. We still feel that the nurse practitioner-physician team approach to primary care practice capitalizes maximally on the skills of the nurse and physician and can bring to patient care a rational system of high quality not easily obtainable in traditional practice patterns.

We would like to acknowledge the many helpful comments and criticisms we have received from practitioners throughout the country. Their willingness to take the time to offer criticism of our work is greatly appreciated. Their suggestions have been quite helpful in our efforts to improve this work. We encourage all who use these guidelines to let us know about errors, points of disagreement, or significant alterations to our position.

A.J.H.
R.A.G.
C.G.P.

Introduction: Use of Patient Care Guidelines

Several fundamental concepts underlie these patient care guidelines and need to be made clear at the outset:

1. A nurse practitioner cannot legally carry out medical practice acts without having a working relationship with a physician who agrees to be ultimately responsible for the medical practice acts of the nurse and to be always available for consultation or referral or both. Normal procedures of *nursing* practice, carried out by the nurse practitioner, are not under the supervision of the physician.
2. The guidelines must be thoroughly reviewed, changed if necessary, and mutually agreed to by the nurse practitioner and physician before they are implemented.
3. The patient care guidelines define the boundaries of the medical practice acts available to the nurse practitioner. If there is no guideline defining a condition and its management, the nurse practitioner must not diagnose or treat the condition without direct physician involvement.
4. The nurse practitioner and responsible physician must assure one another through supervised practice that the nurse practitioner has the knowledge and skills to make the diagnosis contained in the guidelines and to render treatment as outlined. The guidelines are *not* intended to serve as a "cookbook" reference work to assist in making diagnoses. Rather, they are an attempt to codify the knowledge and practices of the nurse and physician.

In settings in which we have had experience, the guidelines cover about 75 percent of the presenting problems of patients seeking primary health care. Obviously in certain settings other conditions may occur more frequently, and the need to develop additional guidelines may arise. Thus, the need to review one's practice and to develop or revise guidelines is constant.

In practice, the guidelines have been used to enable the nurse practitioner legally and ethically to engage in medical practice acts without the physician's personally seeing each patient. In certain settings, the nurse and physician may be geographically separated, as when the nurse practitioner operates a satellite clinic. In this context, the guidelines are often referred to as *standing orders.* The clinical note should contain adequate information to assure anyone reading it that the patient's condition fits the guideline being followed. In practice, the nurse practitioner needs to refer to the guidelines for common conditions only as a check; the condition being managed and the correct procedures for treating it usually are known before the guidelines are checked.

An additional use for the guidelines is a standard of care in medical audit procedures. Effective use of the guidelines in this manner, however, demands that the practitioners being audited have an opportunity to review, discuss, and modify the guidelines *before* any audit begins in order to ensure that they are appropriate standards for the geographic area and the specific practice.

We do not presume to assert that the guidelines we have developed apply immediately everywhere as standards of care. They should simply serve as a point of departure from which to develop guidelines that suit local norms and conditions.

A final word about the format. Originally we experimented with clinical algorithms, or branching logic trees. Although we found these useful in attempting to analzye the clinician's approach to clinical problem solving, we found them unworkable as guides to practice. Experienced, well-trained practitioners simply do not follow the same branching logic in dealing with every patient. The same key observations are made, but not necessarily in the same order. We therefore abandoned that format.

We again wish to emphasize that this is, and should remain, an unfin-ished work. In this regard, we welcome the comments and suggestions of others. We sincerely hope that this book will contribute to the continuing effort to provide improved patient care.

Patient Care Guidelines
for Nurse Practitioners

Use of the Health Maintenance Flow Sheet Age Two Weeks to Seventeen Years

I. Purpose of the health maintenance flow sheet (Fig. 1)

A. To guide the health care provider in recommended health mainte-nance procedures.

B. To serve as a data sheet for recording the results of procedu.

C. To individualize a patient's health maintenance program appropi. ately.

D. To summarize a patient's health maintenance status.

II. General instructions

A. At the patient's first health maintenance visit after registration, the recommended procedures that are appropriate for the patient's age are done; see Age-Specific Health Maintenance Guidelines (Pediatric).

B. The date (month and year) are recorded beside each procedure in the first blank column.

C. The date of the next scheduled assessment is written in the top box of the next column (opposite the heading "Date scheduled").

D. Moving down the column, the boxes of the procedures to be done at the next assessment should be *outlined* by the provider with a red pencil. No other columns are marked in advance, since the purpose of outlining the procedure boxes in each column is to indicate what should be done at or before the next assessment. This can be determined only by what was actually done by the end of the previous assessment.

E. If procedures are done before the next scheduled assessment, the date when they are done and the results are recorded in the red-outlined box.

F. This sequence is repeated at each scheduled assessment. If a patient develops a problem that requires more frequent visits, the reg-

Procedures and Ages						
Assessments: 2 wk; 2, 4, 6, 9, 12, 18 mo; 2, 3, 5, 8, 11, 13, 15, 17 yr	Date scheduled					
	Date seen					
	Age					
	Provider					
Complete history	Date					
Complete examination	Date					
Immunizations (record dates below)						
DPT						
OPV						
MMR						
Hib						
Td						
Tuberculin test if at risk 1, 3, 5, 11, 15 yr	Pos/Neg					
Hematocrit 1, 5, 13 yr	Result					
Urine culture (female) 5, 8 yr	Nl/Abn					
Blood pressure 3 yr and each subsequent visit	Result					
Development Each visit	Nl/Abn/?					
Hearing 6 mo; 1, 3 yr; and each subsequent visit	P/F					
Vision 4 mo; 1, 3 yr; and each subsequent visit	P/F					
Language 2, 3, 5 yr	P/F					
Dental care Each visit						
Counseling: each visit						
Nutrition						
Physical care						
Behavior/psychosocial						
Sex education						
Stimulation						
Safety						
Family planning						
Other						

Figure 1-1. Health maintenance flow sheet (2 weeks to 17 years).

ular medical record—not the health maintenance flow sheet—is used for such extra visits.

G. If an indicated procedure is not done or needs to be repeated, the appropriate box of the next assessment is outlined at each visit until the procedure is done. At that time, a check mark is placed in the box or a result is recorded.

H. The information recorded on the health maintenance flow sheet does not have to be recorded in the regular medical record entry. That entry should contain the interval medical history, whatever physical examination is done, any medication prescribed, and any details that the provider feels will be helpful for future visits (e.g., certain counseling subjects that will need particular emphasis at future visits).

te: Unlike most health maintenance flow sheets, this one is based o. he procedures this particular patient has actually had and on those nee d by the specific date of the next scheduled assessment. By merely look r down the column after the date of a scheduled assessment has passe one can tell what procedures a patient still needs. Thus, audit of heal maintenance status is simplified.

III. Specific cedures

A. **Assess nts.** Record the date the patient was seen, the patient's age, and health care provider's initials. The 2-week assessment is carried o in the home, subsequent ones in the clinic. Enter the date of the xt scheduled assessment in the next column. Note that the assessm m number of assessments that all patients should have. If problems are discovered, more frequent assessments may be needed. These additional assessments are recorded not on this flow sheet but in the medical record. A flow sheet for a specific problem (e.g., urinary tract infection) may be indicated.

B. **Complete history.** The complete health history should include past medical history, family history, social history, and review of systems. An age-specific health questionnaire, which is reviewed with the parent or patient, or both, and commented on in the medical record, is recommended. The history should be taken as soon as possible after registration. The date that it is completed is entered in the appropriate box. At each assessment, an appropriate interval medical history is taken, but it need not be noted on the health maintenance flow sheet.

C. **Complete examination.** A complete physical examination should be performed as soon as possible after registration. Enter the date it is completed in the appropriate box. The extent of subsequent physical examinations, which need not be recorded on the flow sheet, is determined by the age-specific health maintenance guidelines (discussed later in this chapter) and by clinical judgment based on the interval medical history and the patient's age and problem list.

D. **Immunizations.** See Age-Specific Health Maintenance Guidelines (Pediatric) for recommended program. Contraindications should be carefully reviewed before giving any vaccine. Contraindications for all immunizations include acute febrile illness (a minor infection not associated with fever is not a contraindication) and prior adverse reaction to the same or a related vaccine. For precautions and contraindications for DPT vaccine, see Morbidity and Mortality Weekly Report (MMWR) 1985; 34:413–14, 419–21. General contraindications for all live virus vaccines include: (1) immunosuppressive therapy (radiation therapy, corticosteroids, antimetabolites, alkylating agents, and cytotoxic drugs); (2) immunodeficiency disorders; (3) leukemia, lymphoma, or generalized malignancy; (4) pregnancy; and (5) recent (within 8 weeks) immune globulin, plasma, or blood transfusions. Refer to the *Report of the Committee on Infectious Diseases* (the "Red Book") of the American Academy of Pediatrics* for further details. If a patient will need an immunization by the next scheduled assessment, outline the box in the next scheduled assessment column and write in the immunization that will be needed. Place a check mark in the most recently outlined box when immunizations are up to date. A record of the date that each specific immunization is given is entered in the appropriate box in the Procedures column and also on the immunization record card that is given to parents.

E. **Tuberculin test.** The decision to administer this test can depend on the prevalence of tuberculosis in the population. Record the date the test is given and the result as positive (pos) or negative (neg).

F. **Hematocrit.** Record the date the test is done and the hematocrit value (see Table 1-1).

G. **Urine culture.** Record the date the specimen is collected and the result as normal (Nl) or abnormal (Abn). Normal is less than 10,000 organisms per milliliter on a clean midstream specimen. Consult Chapter 9, Urinary Tract Infection (Pediatric), IV, p. 230, if the culture has more than 10,000 organisms per milliliter.

H. **Blood pressure.** Record the date and the blood pressure. Be sure to use a cuff that covers two-thirds of the arm, with the inflatable portion completely encircling the arm. Table 1-2 shows normal blood pressure values.

I. **Development.** The Denver Prescreening Developmental Questionnaire† or a similar, established instrument should be used. Record

---

*This report is revised and published every few years by the American Academy of Pediatrics, P.O. Box 1034, Evanston, Ill. 60204.

†Ladoca Project & Publishing Foundation, Inc., East 51st Avenue & Lincoln Street, Denver, Colo. 80216.

Table 1-1. Minimum normal hematocrit values at different ages

Age	Hematocrit
6 months to 6 years	33
6–14 years	35
Over 14	
Female	36
Male	40

Table 1-2. Maximum normal values of blood pressure recorded in the supine position.

Age (years)	Systolic/diastolic (mm Hg)
0–3	110/65
3–7	120/70
7–10	130/75
10–13	140/80
13–15	
Male	140/80
Female	140/85
Over 15	140/90

the date when the test is done. ⸌ ⸍ults are recorded as normal (Nl), abnormal (Abn), or questionable (?).

J. Hearing. Record the date and the result as pass (P) or fail (F). The following screening tests should be used:

  1. Six to twenty-four months

  a. Parent gives a history of infant's vocalization and response to sound; see Age-Specific Health Maintenance Guidelines (Pediatric).

  b. Infant ceases activity on hearing a conversational voice or orients himself toward the voice, or both.

  c. With the infant held, his attention should be fixed on a visual stimulus. The source of sound should be held 4 feet to one side of the infant's head, out of peripheral vision. The infant should respond to low-pitched (clacker or block and hammer), medium-pitched (squeaky toy), and high-pitched (bell) sounds.

  2. Three to seventeen years. Pure-tone audiometry. For procedure, see *Standards of Child Health Care* (3rd ed.), Evanston, Ill.: American Academy of Pediatrics, 1977, pp. 146–148.

K. Vision. Record the date and the result as pass (P) or fail (F). In addition, record actual visual acuity in the medical record when the Snellen E test is used. The following screening tests should be performed:

1. **Under four years**

   a. Pupil size, shape, and reaction to light.

   b. Ability to follow light.

   c. Ability to pick up small, raisin-sized object (over 9 months of age).

   d. Evidence of strabismus by history, position of light reflection on cornea, and extraocular movements.

   e. Evidence of latent strabismus by cover-uncover test.

2. **Four years and over**

   a. Pupil size, shape, and reaction to light.

   b. Evidence of strabismus by history, position of light reflection on cornea, and extraocular movements.

   c. Evidence of latent strabismus by cover-uncover test.

   d. Snellen E test

      (1) Place the child 20 feet from the well-illuminated chart. Each child is tested on the 20/50, 20/40, 20/30, and 20/20 lines of the chart, using both eyes and each alone, until the criteria for failure are met. A child who wears glasses should be tested with and without the glasses. The examiner should watch for signs of visual problems, such as excessive blinking, squinting, crossed eyes, or tearing.

      (2) Visual acuity is recorded as the lowest line on the chart that is passed. The first number is the distance from the testing chart; the second number is the distance at which the particular line of the chart is readable by the normal person. Criteria for failure are as follows:

         (a) Failure to read more than half the letters of the 20/30 line successfully.

         (b) Difference in acuity between eyes of more than one line—if an entire line is exposed for testing at a time; *or,* difference in acuity between eyes of one line—if only one E is exposed for testing at a time.

         (c) Observation of visual problems by the examiner.

L. Language. For procedures, see Age-Specific Health Maintenance Guidelines (Pediatric). Record the date and the result as pass (P) or fail (F).

M. Dental care. Record date. Teeth and gums should be examined and parents and patient counseled on dental care. See Age-Specific Health Maintenance Guidelines (Pediatric) for details. Patients are referred to a dental service for screening and health education at 3 years of age, or at the time of registration if they are older.

N. Counseling. See Age-Specific Health Maintenance Guidelines (Pediatric) for counseling under each category. Place a check mark in the appropriate box when this has been done.

O. Other. At the bottom of the flow sheet are empty spaces for other procedures that the provider would like to have as part of an individual's health maintenance program.

Age-Specific Health Maintenance Guidelines: Pediatric

Two-Week Home Visit

I. **Provider.** Nurse practitioner.

II. **History**

  A. Review obstetric and newborn hospital record.

  B. Take interval medical history.

III. **Examination.** Inspection of baby completely undressed.

IV. **Procedures.** None.

V. **Dental care**

  A. Content of fluoride in drinking water should be 0.7–1.2 ppm.

  B. If concentration of fluoride in water or water intake is inadequate, supplemental fluoride should be given, in the form of sodium fluoride (Luride) drops, containing 0.125 mg of fluoride per drop.

  1. If water supply has less than 0.3 ppm or baby is breast-fed, give 2 drops per day.

  2. If water supply has 0.3–0.7 ppm and baby consumes some water, give 1 drop per day.

VI. **Counseling**

  A. **Nutrition**

  1. Discuss breast-feeding:

    a. Breast and nipple care.

    b. Normal balanced diet and good fluid intake for mother.

    c. Feeding technique and schedule.

    d. Misconceptions.

      e. Supplemental vitamin D.

      f. Encouragement.

      g. Availability for future counseling if needed.

  2. Discuss bottle-feeding:

      a. Milk formula selection.

      b. Preparation and storage techniques.

      c. Supplemental vitamins if not in formula.

      d. Feeding technique and schedule.

  3. Discuss parents' questions.

B. Physical care

  1. Assess adequacy of physical environment for newborn with appropriate counseling or agency referral, or both, as needed.

  2. Discuss skin care for baby:

      a. Minor and periodic variations in normal skin.

      b. Bathing techniques.

      c. Care of diaper area.

      d. Care of umbilical cord stump.

      e. Clothing (avoid overheating).

  3. Discuss parents' questions.

C. Behavior and psychosocial environment

  1. Assess adequacy of emotional environment:

      a. Postpartum depression. Evaluate available supports, such as father, grandparents, public health nurse, caretaker, day nursery, social worker.

      b. Mother-infant interaction. Was baby wanted? Is it of the desired sex? What are mother's expectations of baby?

      c. Role of father. Evaluate degree of support he can provide and his expectations of baby.

      d. Adjustment of siblings to baby.

  2. Discuss infant behavior and normal variations:

      a. Crying.

      b. Sleeping and breathing patterns.

      c. Bowel movements.

3. Assess appropriateness of concepts of discipline and punishment.

4. Discuss parents' questions.

D. Stimulation. See Infant and Child Stimulation Guidelines, p. 39.

E. Safety. Advise parents on the following safety practices:

1. Use special infant carseat for automobile travel. Parent's lap is *not* safe.

2. Be certain crib meets safety standards of the Consumer Product Safety Commission.

3. Never leave infant without protection to prevent falling from a surface.

4. Never leave infant alone in the bath water.

5. Hot water faucet temperature should be below 130°F to prevent accidental burns.

6. Protect from young siblings and pets.

F. Family planning.

G. Other topics, based on parents' concerns.

VII. Follow-up

A. Explain the purpose of health maintenance visits. Review flow sheet with parents.

B. Give clinic telephone number.

C. Schedule first appointment.

D. Leave medical questionnaire with parent to be completed just before first clinic visit and brought to clinic.

E. Emphasize availability of health care and counseling before scheduled clinic visit, if needed.

Two-Month Clinic Visit

I. **Provider.** Physician.

II. **History**

A. Review neonatal hospital summary.

B. Review record of 2-week home visit.

C. Take dietary history.

D. Take development history.

    E. Take family medical history.

    F. Take social history.

    G. Review systems.

III. Examination

    A. Measurements (record on growth chart):

        1. Weight.

        2. Length.

        3. Head circumference.

    B. Complete physical examination.

IV. Procedures*

    A. Immunizations, after reviewing contraindications and discussing side effects:

        1. Diphtheria-pertussis-tetanus vaccine.

        2. Oral polio vaccine (trivalent).

    B. Developmental appraisal.

V. Dental care. Give supplemental fluoride, if necessary (see Two-Week Home Visit, **V,** p. 7).

VI. Counseling

    A. Nutrition

        1. Review milk formula or breast-feeding, or both.

        2. Review preparation and storage techniques.

        3. Discuss the adequacy of milk alone as the source of nutrition until at least 4 months of age.

        4. Give supplemental vitamins if not in formula or Vitamin D if the mother is breast-feeding.

        5. Discuss iron requirements:

            a. Breast milk will supply sufficient iron for full-term babies.

            b. Iron-fortified formula.

              or

            c. Ferrous sulfate (Fer-In-Sol) drops (15 mg elemental iron per 0.6 ml). For infants weighing 4–7 kg (8–14 lb), give 0.3 ml once a day in water or fruit juice. For infants weighing more

---

*See Use of the Health Maintenance Flow Sheet, pp. 1–7, for details.

than 7 kg (more than 14 lb) and all premature babies, give 0.6 ml once a day.

    6. Discuss parents' questions.

B. Physical care

    1. Discuss baby's response to common respiratory and gastrointestinal illnesses, home management, and indications for seeking medical care.

    2. Discuss parents' questions.

C. Behavior and psychosocial environment

    1. Assess adequacy of emotional environment, with counseling when appropriate:

        a. Mother-infant interaction: Observe for overprotectiveness, lack of warmth toward baby, signs of maternal depression.

        b. Role of father.

        c. Role of siblings—management of sibling rivalry.

        d. Role of extended family and support systems (grandparents, friends).

    2. Discuss behavior changes expected before next visit.

    3. Discuss parents' questions.

D. Stimulation. See Infant and Child Stimulation Guidelines, p. 39.

E. Safety. Advise parents on the following safety practices:

    1. Use special infant carseat for automobile travel. Parent's lap is *not* safe.

    2. Be certain crib meets safety standards of the Consumer Product Safety Commission.

    3. Never leave infant without protection to prevent falling from a surface.

    4. Never leave infant alone in bath water.

    5. Hot water faucet temperature should be below 130°F to prevent accidental burns.

    6. Keep objects or toys that are sharp, breakable, ingestible, or that have cords away from baby.

    7. Protect from young siblings and pets.

F. Family planning

G. Other topics, based on parents' concerns.

VII. Follow-up. In 2 months, or sooner if necessary.

Four-Month Clinic Visit

I. Provider. Nurse practitioner.

II. History. Interval history.

III. Examination

    A. Measurements (record on growth chart):

        1. Weight.

        2. Length.

        3. Head circumference.

    B. Inspection of baby completely undressed.

    C. Extent of further examination is based on interval medical history and patient's problem list.

IV. Procedures*

    A. Immunizations, after reviewing contraindications and discussing side effects.

        1. Diphtheria-pertussis-tetanus vaccine.

        2. Oral polio vaccine (trivalent).

    B. Developmental appraisal.

    C. Vision screening.

V. Dental care

    A. Give supplemental fluoride, if necessary (see Two-Week Home Visit, **V**, p. 7).

    B. Discuss teething and the use of teething toys and hard crackers.

VI. Counseling

    A. Nutrition

        1. Continue milk formula or breast-feeding, or both.

        2. Discuss gradual introduction of solid foods.

        3. Give supplemental vitamins if not in formula or if the mother is breast-feeding.

        4. Discuss iron requirements:

            a. Breast-feeding plus iron-fortified cereal by six months of age.

*See Use of the Health Maintenance Flow Sheet, pp. 1-7, for details.

b. Iron-fortified formula

or

c. Ferrous sulfate (Fer-In-Sol) drops (15 mg elemental iron per 0.6 ml). For infants weighing 7 mg or less (14 lb or less), give 0.3 ml once a day in water or fruit juice. For infants weighing over 7 kg (over 14 lb) and all premature babies, give 0.6 ml once a day.

5. Discuss parents' questions.

B. Physical care

1. Review baby's response to common respiratory and gastrointestinal illnesses, home management, and indications for seeking medical care.

2. Discuss parents' questions.

C. Behavior and psychosocial environment

1. Assess mother-infant interaction and role of father.

2. Discuss alternative caretakers to allow mother time free from baby. Discuss attitude toward mother's returning to work and using day care.

3. Discuss behavior changes expected before next visit.

4. Discuss parents' questions.

D. Stimulation. See Infant and Child Stimulation Guidelines, p. 39.

E. Safety. Advise parents on the following safety practices:

1. Use special infant carseat for automobile travel. Parent's lap is *not* safe.

2. Be certain crib meets safety standards of the Consumer Product Safety Commission.

3. Discuss infant's increasing mobility and risk of rolling off surfaces. Keep crib sides up.

4. Never leave infant alone in bath water.

5. Hot water faucet temperature should be below 130°F to prevent accidental burns.

6. Keep objects or toys which are sharp, breakable, ingestible, or which have cords away from baby.

7. Protect from young siblings and pets.

F. Other topics, based on parents' concerns.

VII. Follow-up. In 2 months, or sooner if necessary.

Six-Month Clinic Visit

I. Provider. Nurse practitioner.

II. History. Interval medical history.

III. Examination

    A. Measurements (record on growth chart):

        1. Weight.

        2. Length.

        3. Head circumference.

    B. Complete physical examination.

IV. Procedures*

    A. Immunizations, after reviewing contraindications and discussing side effects.

        1. Diphtheria-pertussis-tetanus vaccine.

        2. Oral polio vaccine (trivalent).

    B. Developmental appraisal

    C. Hearing screening. Ask parents these questions:

        1. Does your baby stir or awaken when sleeping quietly and some-one talks or makes a loud noise nearby? (The baby does not have to do this all the time, but should occasionally.)

        2. Does your baby sometimes start or jump when there is a very loud noise, such as a cough, dog bark, or object dropped?

V. Dental care

    A. Give supplemental fluoride, if necessary (see Two-Week Home Visit, **V,** p. 7).

    B. Discuss teething and the use of teething toys and hard crackers for biting if not done at previous visit.

    C. To prevent caries, tell parents not to leave a nursing bottle in the crib with the baby after teeth have erupted.

VI. Counseling

    A. Nutrition

        1. Continue milk formula or breast-feeding, or both.

        2. Watch for excessive weight gain.

*See Use of the Health Maintenance Flow Sheet, pp. 1–7, for details.

3. Discuss importance of basic food groups and of avoiding non-nutritious sugared commercial foods.

4. Discuss need for supplemental vitamins if not in formula or vitamin D if breast-feeding.

5. Discuss iron requirements:

   a. Iron-fortified formula

      or

   b. Ferrous sulfate (Fer-In-Sol) drops (15 mg elemental iron per 0.6 ml) 0.6 ml once a day in water or fruit juice

      and, for breast- and bottle-fed infants,

   c. Iron fortified cereals and iron-containing foods.

6. Discuss parents' questions.

B. Physical care

1. Review parental management of illnesses occurring since previous visit.

2. Discuss parents' questions.

C. Behavior and psychosocial environment

1. Assess maternal-infant interaction and role of father.

2. Discuss parents' attitude toward discipline. Emphasize that the baby is too young to "behave."

3. Discuss adjustment of siblings to baby.

4. Discuss stranger anxiety—baby-sitter should be familiar to the baby before parents leave.

5. Discuss parents' questions.

D. Stimulation. See Infant and Child Stimulation Guidelines, p. 39.

E. Safety. Advise parents on the following safety practices:

1. Use special infant carseat for automobile travel. Parent's lap is *not* safe.

2. Be certain crib meets safety standards of the Consumer Product Safety Commission.

3. Never leave infant alone in bath water or near a pool.

4. Hot water faucet temperature should be below 130°F to prevent accidental burns.

5. Prepare house for infant's increasing mobility:

   a. Cover electric outlets with plug guards.

b. Disconnect all cords to appliances when not in use.

c. Keep sharp, breakable, or ingestible objects out of reach, of floor and low tables.

d. Avoid small, hard foods that could be aspirated into airway (e.g., peanuts).

e. Lock medicines, cleaning materials, and poisons away and out of reach [review the use of syrup of ipecac as described in Chapter 2, Ingestions and Poisonings (Pediatric), **VI.E, p** 81].

f. Keep handles of pots turned away from reach.

g. Keep hot food containers out of reach on tables, and do not use tablecloths that can be pulled down.

h. Put gate across top of stairs.

i. Place guards in front of space heaters, heating stoves, and radiators.

j. Keep screens in open windows.

k. Keep child in enclosed space when outdoors and not in the company of an adult.

F. **Other topics,** based on parents' concerns.

VII. **Follow-up.** In 3 months, or sooner if necessary.

Nine-Month Clinic Visit

I. **Provider.** Nurse practitioner.

II. **History.** Interval medical history.

III. **Examination**

A. Measurements (record on growth chart):

1. Weight.

2. Length.

3. Head circumference.

B. Inspection of baby completely undressed.

C. Extent of further examination is based on interval history and patient's problem list.

IV. **Procedures***

*See Use of the Health Maintenance Flow Sheet, pp. 1–7, for details.

   A. Review flow sheet to be certain that procedures indicated at previous visits have been completed.

   B. Developmental appraisal.

V. Dental care

   A. Examine teeth.

   B. Give supplemental fluoride, if necessary (see Two-Week Home Visit, **V**, p. 7).

   C. To prevent caries, tell parents not to leave a nursing bottle in the crib with the baby.

   D. Tell parents to clean teeth with gauze pad once a day.

VI. Counseling

   A. Nutrition

   1. Continue milk formula or breast-feeding, or both.

   2. Review diet. Counsel on importance of basic food groups and of avoiding nonnutritious sugared commercial foods. Consider family preferences and economic factors.

   3. Give supplemental vitamins if not in formula or vitamin D if breast-feeding.

   4. Discuss iron requirements:

   a. Iron-fortified formula

   or

   b. Ferrous sulfate (Fer-In-Sol) drops (15 mg elemental iron per 0.6 ml) 0.6 ml once a day in water or fruit juice

   and, for breast and bottle-fed infants,

   c. Iron-fortified cereals and iron-containing foods.

   5. Discuss management of food preferences and possible decrease in appetite.

   B. Physical care

   1. Review parental management of illnesses occurring since previous visit.

   2. Discuss parents' questions.

   C. Behavior and psychosocial environment

   1. Assess family's response to annoying behavior. Help parents to realize that baby is not yet able to be disciplined.

   2. Discuss stranger and separation anxiety.

3. Discuss child's desire to use spoon and cup for feeding and ex pected messiness.

4. Discuss parents' questions and expectations of baby.

D. Stimulation. See Infant and Child Stimulation Guidelines, p. 39.

E. Safety. Advise parents on the following safety practices:

1. Use special infant carseat for automobile travel. Parent's lap i *not* safe.

2. Be certain crib meets safety standards of the Consumer Produc Safety Commission.

3. Never leave infant alone in bath water or near a pool.

4. Hot water faucet temperature should be below 130°F to preven accidental burns.

5. Prepare house for infant's increasing mobility:

   a. Cover electric outlets with plug guards.

   b. Disconnect all cords to appliances when not in use.

   c. Keep sharp, breakable, or ingestible objects out of reach, of floor and low tables.

   d. Avoid small, hard foods that could be aspirated into airwa (e.g., peanuts).

   e. Lock medicines, cleaning materials, and poisons away an out of reach [review the use of syrup of ipecac as describe in Chapter 2, Ingestions and Poisonings (Pediatric), **VI.E**, p 81].

   f. Keep handles of pots turned away from reach.

   g. Keep hot food containers out of reach on tables and do no use tablecloths that can be pulled down.

   h. Put gate across top of stairs.

   i. Place guards in front of space heaters, heating stoves, an radiators.

   j. Keep screens in open windows.

   k. Keep child in enclosed space when outdoors and not in th company of an adult.

F. Other topics, based on parents' concerns.

VII. Follow-up. In 3 months, or sooner if necessary.

Twelve-Month Clinic Visit

I. **Provider.** Physician.

II. **History.** Interval medical history.

III. **Examination**

    A. Measurements (record on growth chart):

        1. Weight.

        2. Length.

        3. Head circumference.

    B. Complete physical examination.

IV. **Procedures***

    A. Hematocrit determination (normal is greater than 32%).

    B. Developmental appraisal.

    C. Hearing screening. Ask parents the following questions:

        1. Does your baby turn his head in any direction to find an interesting sound or the person speaking?

        2. Does your baby stir or awaken when sleeping quietly and someone talks or makes a loud sound nearby?

    D. Vision screening.

    E. **Tuberculin skin test,** depending on the prevalence of tuberculosis in the population.

V. **Dental care**

    A. Examine teeth.

    B. Give supplemental fluoride, if necessary (see Two-Week Home Visit, **V**, p. 7).

    C. To prevent caries, tell parents not to leave a nursing bottle in the crib with the baby.

    D. Discuss rationale for avoiding frequent snacks or sugar-containing foods.

    E. Remind parents to clean teeth with soft toothbrush or gauze pad once a day.

VI. **Counseling**

---

*See Use of the Health Maintenance Flow Sheet, pp. 1–7, for details.

A. Nutrition

1. Try to keep milk intake under 20 ounces if a balanced diet is available.

2. Review diet. Counsel again, if necessary, on importance of basic food groups and of avoiding nonnutritious sugared commercial foods. Consider family preferences and economic factors.

3. Continue iron-fortified formula *or* ferrous sulfate (Fer-In-Sol) drops (15 mg elemental iron per 0.6 ml), 0.6 ml once a day in water or juice.

4. If necessary, discuss again management of food preferences and possible decrease in appetite.

B. Physical care

1. Review parental management of illness occurring since previous visit.

2. Discuss parents' questions.

C. Behavior and psychosocial environment

1. Discuss parents' concept of acceptable behavior and discipline and their expectations.

2. Discuss adjustment of family to curiosity, mobility, and negativism of baby and their tolerance of noise from baby and siblings.

3. Discuss management of separations.

4. Explore parents' concept of toilet training.

5. Discuss child's progress toward drinking mainly from cup.

6. Discuss parents' questions.

D. Stimulation. See Infant and Child Stimulation Guidelines, p. 39.

E. Safety. See Nine-Month Clinic Visit, VI.E, p. 18.

F. Other topics, based on parents' concerns.

VII. Follow-up. Measles-mumps-rubella vaccine to be given at age 15 months. Routine health maintenance visit in 6 months, or sooner if necessary.

Eighteen-Month Clinic Visit

I. Provider. Nurse practitioner.

II. History

A. Interval medical history.

B. Review and revision of family and social history.

III. Examination

A. Measurements (record on growth chart):

1. Weight.

2. Length.

3. Head circumference.

B. Inspection of baby completely undressed.

C. Extent of further examination is based on interval history and patient's problem list.

IV. Procedures*

A. Immunizations, after reviewing contraindications and discussing side effects.

1. Diphtheria-pertussis-tetanus vaccine.

2. Oral polio vaccine (trivalent).

3. Hemophilus influenzae type b (Hib) vaccine, if attending day care. Otherwise give at 2 years of age.

B. Developmental appraisal.

V. Dental care

A. Examine teeth.

B. Give supplemental fluoride, if necessary (see Two-Week Home Visit, **V**, p. 7).

C. Discuss rationale for avoiding frequent snacks of sugar-containing foods.

D. Remind parents to clean teeth with soft toothbrush or gauze pad twice a day.

VI. Counseling

A. Nutrition

1. Review diet. Counsel again, if necessary, on importance of basic food groups and of avoiding nonnutritious sugared commercial foods. Consider family preferences and economic factors.

2. Limit milk intake to 2–3 glasses per day if a balanced diet is available.

3. Discuss progress of self-feeding.

4. Discuss parents' questions.

*See Use of the Health Maintenance Flow Sheet, pp. 1–7, for details.

B. Physical care

1. Review parental management of illnesses occurring since previous visit.

2. Discuss parents' questions.

C. Behavior and psychosocial environment

1. Discuss adjustment of family to baby's negativism, and possible frustration of parents' expectations of baby.

2. Discuss discipline and limit setting. Encourage parents to use substitution and positive reinforcement rather than physical punishment.

3. Discuss management of separation from mother.

4. Discuss toilet training and variations in normal patterns.

5. Discuss sleep problems (e.g., night terrors, desire to sleep in parents' room).

6. Discuss parents' questions.

D. Stimulation. See Infant and Child Stimulation Guidelines, p. 39.

E. Safety. Review hazards and precautions discussed at previous visit (see Nine-Month Clinic Visit, **VI.E**, p. 18).

F. Other topics, based on parents' concerns.

VII. Follow-up. In 6 months, or sooner if necessary.

Two-Year Clinic Visit

I. Provider. Nurse practitioner.

II. History. Interval medical history.

III. Examination

A. Measurements (record on growth chart):

1. Weight.

2. Length.

3. Head circumference.

B. Complete physical examination.

IV. Procedures*

A. Immunizations. Hemophilus influenzae type b (Hib) vaccine.

B. Developmental appraisal.

---

*See Use of the Health Maintenance Flow Sheet, pp. 1–7, for details.

C. Hearing screening.

  1. Does baby point to at least one part of the body (eyes, feet, etc.) when you ask, without seeing your lips?

  2. Does baby point to the right picture when asked, without seeing your lips, "Where's the cat [dog, man, horse, etc]?"

  3. Does baby give you a toy or put an object on a table or chair when asked, without seeing your lips?

  Note: Baby may pass this test by observation of examiner or report of parent. Since this test evaluates more than just hearing function, failure requires further evaluation of other aspects of development as well.

D. Language screening. Ask parent what words the child uses regularly to denote specific objects, persons, or actions. This procedure is passed if parent reports child has three words other than *Dada* and *Mama*. Words do not have to be intelligible, but they must be specific.

V. Dental care

  A. Examine teeth.

  B. Give supplemental fluoride, if necessary.

   1. Content of fluoride in drinking water should be 0.7–1.2 ppm.

   2. If concentration in water or water intake is inadequate, sodium fluoride (Luride) drops, containing 0.125 mg of fluoride per drop, should be given:

     a. If water supply has less than 0.3 ppm, give 4 drops per day.

     b. If water supply has 0.3–0.7 ppm, give 2 drops per day.

  C. Discuss rationale for avoiding frequent snacks of sugar-containing foods.

  D. Remind parents to clean teeth with toothbrush or gauze pad twice a day.

  E. Refer to dental services before age 3, even if teeth appear normal.

VI. Counseling

  A. Nutrition

   1. Review diet. Counsel again, if necessary, on importance of basic food groups, of avoiding nonnutritious sugared commercial foods, and of limiting milk to 2–3 glasses per day if a balanced diet is available. Consider family preferences and economic factors.

   2. Discuss progress of self-feeding.

   3. Discuss parents' questions.

B. Physical care

1. Review parental management of illnesses occurring since previous visit.

2. Discuss parents' questions.

C. Behavior and psychosocial environment

1. Discuss parents' concepts of normal behavior and limits. Discuss the fact that child understands "No" before inner controls are available to obey.

2. Discuss discipline and use of substitution and positive reinforcement instead of physical punishment.

3. Discuss beginning of toilet training. Encourage independence in toileting when day control is achieved.

4. Discuss management of separation from mother.

5. Discuss sleep problems.

6. Discuss parents' questions.

D. Stimulation. See Infant and Child Stimulation Guidelines, p. 39.

E. Safety. Advise parents on the following safety practices:

1. Lock doors where danger of falling exists (e.g., cellar stairs).

2. Lock up sharp or electrical tools.

3. Check driveway, while outside automobile, before backing up.

4. Lock all car doors.

5. Never leave child unrestrained in cargo section of station wagon.

6. Put matches out of reach.

7. See also Nine-Month Clinic Visit, **VI.E**, p. 18.

VII. Follow-up. In 1 year, or sooner if necessary.

Three-Year Clinic Visit

I. Provider. Nurse practitioner.

II. History

A. Interval medical history.

B. Review and revision of family and social history.

III. Examination

A. Measurements (record on growth chart):

1. Weight.
2. Length.

B. Complete physical examination.

IV. Procedures*

A. Tuberculin skin test, depending on prevalence of tuberculosis in the population.

B. Blood pressure (normal is less than 120/70 mm Hg in the supine position).

C. Developmental appraisal.

D. Hearing screening.

E. Vision screening.

F. Language screening. This test is passed if child makes sentences of three or more words and speech is largely intelligible to strangers.

V. Dental care

A. Examine teeth.

B. Give supplemental fluoride, if necessary (see Two-Year Clinic Visit, **V.B**, p. 23).

C. Discuss rationale for avoiding frequent snacks of sugar-containing foods.

D. Remind parents to brush child's teeth twice a day with anticariogenic toothpaste.

E. Refer if patient was not seen by dental service within the previous year.

VI. Counseling

A. Nutrition

1. Review diet. Counsel again, if necessary, on importance of basic food groups and of avoiding nonnutritious sugared commercial foods. Consider family preferences and economic factors.

2. Discuss possibility of periods of decreased appetite.

3. Explain that eating patterns are influenced by other family members.

4. Discuss parents' questions.

B. Physical care

*See Use of the Health Maintenance Flow Sheet, pp. 1–7, for details.

    1. Review parental management of illnesses occurring since previous visit.

    2. Discuss parents' questions.

C. Behavior and psychosocial environment

    1. Discuss balance between need for independence and realistic discipline, guidance, and limits.

    2. Discuss need for social interaction with peers.

    3. Discuss normal early childhood fears (e.g., body injury), imagination (which is different from lying), and curiosity.

    4. Discuss value and characteristics of good nursery school and day care. Assist family in identifying a program, if desired.

    5. Discuss sibling rivalry if new baby is due or has arrived.

    6. Discuss normal lapses in bladder and bowel control. Issue is not to be made of these with child.

    7. Discuss parents' questions.

D. Sex education (age 3–5 years)

    1. Explore parents' concept of normal psychosexual development in preschool child.

    2. Discuss sexual identity and common questions asked by children, including masturbation and sexual curiosity about other children's anatomy.

E. Stimulation. See Infant and Child Stimulation Guidelines, p. 39.

F. Safety. Advise parents on the following safety practices:

    1. Lock doors where danger of falling exists (e.g., cellar).

    2. Place screens or guards over windows.

    3. Place guards in front of all space heaters, heating stoves, and radiators.

    4. Lock up sharp or electrical tools and firearms.

    5. Lock up poisons and medications [review the use of syrup of ipecac as described in Chapter 2, Ingestions and Poisonings (Pediatric), **VI.E**, p. 81].

    6. Teach child to watch out for moving automobiles in driveways and streets.

    7. Use special young child's carseat for automobile. Shoulder belt may be used. Never leave child unrestrained in cargo section of station wagon.

    8. Lock all car doors.

9. Never allow child to swim or wade in water without adult supervision.

G. Other topics, based on parents' concerns.

VII. Follow-up. In 2 years, or sooner if necessary.

Five-Year Clinic Visit

I. Provider. Nurse practitioner.

II. History

A. Interval medical history, including complete review of systems.

B. Review and revision of family and social history.

III. Examination

A. Measurements (record on growth chart):

1. Weight.

2. Length.

B. Complete physical examination.

IV. Procedures*

A. Immunizations, after reviewing contraindications and discussing side effects.

1. Diphtheria-pertussis-tetanus vaccine.

2. Oral polio vaccine (trivalent).

3. Be certain child has had measles-mumps-rubella vaccine.

B. Tuberculin skin test, depending on the prevalence of tuberculosis in the population.

C. Hematocrit determination (normal is 33% or greater).

D. Urine culture (girls only).

E. Blood pressure (normal is less than 120/70 mm Hg in the supine position).

F. Developmental appraisal.

G. Hearing screening.

H. Vision screening.

I. Language screening. This test is failed if child does any of the following:

*See Use of the Health Maintenance Flow Sheet, pp. 1–7, for details.

    1. Often substitutes easy for difficult sounds (e.g., *wabbit*).

    2. Constantly drops word endings.

    3. Stutters or stammers.

    4. Speaks in a monotonous voice.

    5. Speaks in a voice that is excessively loud or inaudible.

    6. Speaks with hypernasality or hyponasality.

V. Dental care

    A. Examine teeth.

    B. If water supply has less than 0.7 ppm of fluoride, prescribe 1 tablet per day of sodium fluoride (Luride Lozi-Tabs, which releases 1 mg of fluoride per tablet).

    C. Discuss rationale for avoiding frequent snacks of sugar-containing foods.

    D. Remind patient to brush teeth twice a day with anticariogenic toothpaste.

    E. Refer if patient was not seen by dental service within previous year.

VI. Counseling (age 5–8 years)

A. Nutrition

    1. Discuss parents' anxieties about eating problems. Remind them to encourage child's independence, that is, have nutritious foods available but allow child to choose amount and kind of food for his own plate. Reassure parents with growth chart if they are concerned about adequate intake.

    2. Emphasize importance of breakfast, especially when child is going to school all day.

    3. Discuss nutritious after-school snacks.

    4. Encourage parents not to focus on *strict* table manners. Mealtime should be enjoyable for family.

    5. Discuss parents' questions.

B. Physical care

    1. Review parental management of illnesses occurring since previous visit.

    2. Discuss importance of adequate sleep and consistent sleep routine.

    3. Discuss teaching child personal hygiene.

    4. Discuss parents' questions.

C. Behavior and psychosocial environment

1. Discuss preparing child for separation and independence associated with attending school. Assess parental concerns.

2. Discuss importance of regular school attendance.

3. Discuss importance of parent-teacher relationship and periodic meetings.

4. Discuss importance of peer acceptance and need for praise.

5. Discuss the worries and fears common in young school-age children (e.g., death, competition with peers, parental marital conflict, need to achieve). Discuss signs of excessive stress and availability of health care provider for counseling, if needed.

6. Discuss parents' expectations of child (e.g., chores, self-discipline, handling of anger). Are they realistic?

7. Discuss potential problems with teacher after obtaining parental permission.

D. Sex education

1. Explore parents' preparedness for potential questions.

2. Encourage parents to be aware of the scope of sex education programs in school.

E. Stimulation. Parents should be encouraged to do the following:

1. Converse with child regularly. Listen to child and encourage expression of thoughts.

2. Read to child and have child read to them.

3. Be sure child can dress completely.

4. Provide pencil, crayons, paper, paints, and scissors.

5. Show interest in child's schoolwork and provide encouragement.

6. Teach child responsible use of money.

7. Review television-viewing habits. Encourage balanced selective viewing of educational and entertaining programs.

F. Safety. Parents should be encouraged to do the following:

1. Teach child to watch for moving automobiles, especially at intersections. Teach traffic signals and rules.

2. Teach bicycle techniques, traffic rules for bicycles, and warn of danger from automobiles.

3. Teach child swimming skills. Never allow child to swim without adult supervision.

4. Discuss fire prevention in the home with the child.

5. Lock up firearms.

6. Do not allow dangerous tools to be used without supervision.

7. Have child and entire family use seat belts for automobile safety. Lock all car doors. Do not allow child to ride in cargo section of station wagon.

G. Other topics, based on parents' concerns.

VII. Follow-up. In 3 years, or sooner if necessary.

Eight-Year Clinic Visit

I. Provider. Nurse practitioner.

II. History

A. Interval medical history, including complete review of systems.

B. Review and revision of family and social history.

III. Examination

A. Measurements (record on growth chart):

1. Weight.

2. Height.

B. Complete physical examination.

IV. Procedures*

A. Review immunization record.

B. Blood pressure (normal is less than 130/75 mm Hg in the supine position).

C. Hearing screening.

D. Vision screening.

E. Urine culture (girls only).

V. Dental care

A. Examine teeth.

B. Give supplemental fluoride, if necessary (see Five-Year Clinic Visit, **V.B**, p. 28).

C. Discuss rationale for avoiding frequent snacks of sugar-containing foods.

*See Use of the Health Maintenance Flow Sheet, pp. 1–7, for details.

D. Remind patient to brush teeth twice a day with anticariogenic toothpaste and to floss once a day.

E. Refer if patient was not seen by dental service within previous year.

VI. Counseling (age 8–11 years)

A. Nutrition

1. Review diet. Counsel again, if necessary, on importance of basic food groups and of avoiding nonnutritious sugared commercial foods. Consider family preferences and economic factors.

2. Emphasize importance of breakfast, especially when child is going to school all day.

3. Discuss nutritious after-school snacks.

4. Discuss parents' questions.

B. Physical care

1. Review parental management of illnesses occurring since previous visit.

2. Discuss importance of adequate sleep.

3. Discuss parents' questions.

C. Behavior and psychosocial environment

1. Discuss school adjustment and progress with child and parents.

2. Discuss problems with teacher after obtaining parental permission.

3. Discuss importance of parent-teacher relationship and periodic meetings.

4. Explore peer relationships and involvement in group activities (e.g., scouts, religious groups, summer camp, summer recreational programs).

5. Discuss child's interpersonal relationships with siblings and with parents.

6. Discuss parents' and child's attitudes toward responsibilities (e.g., chores, neatness, monetary allowance).

7. Pursue child's as well as parents' concerns.

D. Sex education

1. Discuss parents' response to questions raised by child since previous visit.

2. Encourage parents to be aware of the scope of sex education program in school and to complement it as appropriate.

      3. Discuss possibility of menarche before next visit and parents' plans for discussion with daughter.

      4. Discuss parents' concerns.

  E. Stimulation. Parents should be encouraged to do the following:

      1. Converse with child regularly. Listen to child and encourage expression of thoughts.

      2. Show interest in child's schoolwork.

      3. Provide child with quiet area with as much privacy as possible.

      4. Encourage application of skills learned at school, including the following:

        a. Reading—encourage use of library.

        b. Mathematics—assist child in planning use of money.

        c. Art, music, woodworking—provide child with simple equipment as desired.

      5. Review television-viewing habits. Encourage balanced selective viewing of educational and entertaining programs.

  F. Safety. Parents should be encouraged to do the following:

      1. Teach child the rules of pedestrian and cycling safety.

      2. Encourage development of swimming, water, and boating safety skills. Never allow child to swim without adult supervision.

      3. Discuss fire prevention in home and use of telephone for emergencies.

      4. Lock up firearms.

      5. Do not allow electrical tools to be used without supervision.

      6. Have child and entire family use seat belts for automobile safety. Lock all car doors.

  G. Other topics, based on parents' concerns.

VII. Follow-up. In 3 years, or sooner if necessary.

Eleven-Year Clinic Visit

  I. Provider. Nurse practitioner.

 II. History

  A. Interval medical history, including complete review of systems.

  B. Review and revision of family and social history.

III. Examination

   A. Measurements (record on growth chart):

      1. Weight.

      2. Height.

   B. Complete physical examination.

IV. Procedures*

   A. Review immunization record.

   B. Tuberculin skin test, depending on the prevalence of tuberculosis in the population.

   C. Blood pressure (normal is less than 140/80 mm Hg in the supine position).

   D. Hearing screening.

   E. Vision screening.

V. Dental care

   A. Examine teeth.

   B. Give supplemental fluoride, if necessary (see Five-Year Clinic Visit, **V.B**, p. 28).

   C. Discuss rationale for avoiding frequent snacks or sugar-containing foods.

   D. Remind patient to brush teeth twice a day with anticariogenic toothpaste and to floss once a day.

   E. Refer if patient was not seen by dental service within previous year.

VI. Counseling

   A. Nutrition

      1. Review diet. Counsel parents and child, if necessary, on importance of basic food groups and of avoiding nonnutritious sugared commercial foods. Consider family preferences and economic factors.

      2. Emphasize importance of breakfast, especially when child is going to school all day.

      3. Discuss nutritious after-school snacks.

      4. Discuss parents' and child's questions.

   B. Physical care

      1. Review parental management of illnesses occurring since previous visit.

      2. Discuss importance of adequate sleep and exercise.

*See Use of the Health Maintenance Flow Sheet, pp. 1–7, for details.

   3. Discuss with patient physical changes associated with puberty and the wide variation in time of onset.

   4. Discuss skin care relative to acne.

   5. Discuss parents' and child's questions.

C. Behavior and psychosocial environment

   1. Discuss school adjustment and progress with child and parents. Assess degree of parental involvement and concern.

   2. Discuss problems with school personnel after obtaining parental permission.

   3. Discuss importance of parent-teacher relationship and periodic meetings.

   4. Discuss attitudes of parents and child toward school, achievement, and long-range plans. Are they realistic?

   5. Explore peer relationships and involvement in group activities (e.g., scouts, YMCA or YWCA, religious groups, summer camp, summer recreational programs).

   6. Discuss with parents normal increased desire for independence combined with need for consistent limits and someone who will *listen* to child's concerns.

   7. Discuss child's interpersonal relationships with siblings and parents.

   8. Discuss parents' and child's attitudes toward responsibilities (e.g., chores, neatness, monetary allowance).

   9. Assess and discuss patient's and parents' attitudes toward alcohol, tobacco, and drugs. Counsel as appropriate.

   10. Pursue child's and parents' concerns.

D. Sex education

   1. Discuss parents' response to questions raised by child since previous visit.

   2. Discuss child's understanding of menarche and parents' plans for discussion with daughter.

   3. Discuss variable increase in interest in opposite sex.

   4. Discuss with parents the normal child's concerns and need for sex education, especially girls who mature early. Counsel patient as needed and desired by parents in mechanisms of pregnancy and high-risk relationships. Plan another visit for counseling in this area before next health maintenance visit (age 13), if appropriate. Emphasize to patient and parents your availability.

   E. Safety. Parents should be encouraged to do the following:

    1. Reinforce the rules of pedestrian and cycling safety.

    2. Encourage development of swimming, water, and boating safety skills. Never allow child to swim alone.

    3. Discuss fire prevention in the home and use of telephone for emergencies.

    4. If firearms are available, instruct child in safe use.

    5. Have child and entire family use seat belts for automobile safety. Lock all car doors.

   F. Other topics, based on parents' concerns.

VII. Follow-up. In 2 years, or sooner as needed.

Thirteen- and Fifteen-Year Clinic Visits

  I. Provider. Nurse practitioner.

 II. History

   A. Interval medical history, including complete review of systems.

   B. Review and revision of family and social history.

III. Examination

   A. Measurements (record on growth chart):

    1. Weight.

    2. Height.

   B. Complete physical examination.

IV. Procedures*

   A. Immunizations

    1. Review immunization record.

    2. Tetanus-diphtheria toxoid (adult type-Td), if 10 years have elapsed since previous booster.

   B. Tuberculin skin test at age 15, depending on the prevalence of tuberculosis in the population.

   C. Hematocrit determination at age 13 (normal is greater than 33%).

   D. Blood pressure (normal is less than 140/80 mm Hg for males and less than 140/85 mm Hg for females, in the supine position).

   E. Hearing screening.

*See Use of the Health Maintenance Flow Sheet, pp. 1–7, for details.

   F. Vision screening.

V. Dental care

   A. Examine teeth.

   B. Discuss rationale for avoiding frequent snacks of sugar-containing foods.

   C. Remind patient to brush teeth twice a day with anticariogenic toothpaste and to floss once a day.

   D. Refer if patient was not seen by dental service within previous year.

VI. Counseling (age 13–15 years). Nurse practitioner should meet separately with patient and parents.

   A. Nutrition

   1. Review diet. Counsel patient and parents again, if necessary, on importance of basic food groups. Consider family preferences and economic factors.

   2. Emphasize importance of breakfast, especially when patient is going to school all day.

   3. Discuss nutritious after-school snacks.

   4. Discuss patient's and parents' questions.

   B. Physical care

   1. Review home management of illnesses occurring since previous visit.

   2. Discuss importance of adequate sleep and exercise.

   3. Discuss patient's and parents' questions about physical changes associated with puberty.

   4. Discuss skin care relative to acne.

   5. Discuss patient's and parents' questions.

   C. Behavior and psychosocial environment

   1. Discuss school adjustment and progress with patient and parents.

   2. Discuss problems with school personnel after obtaining permission.

   3. Emphasize practical importance of school relative to careers and employment, if necessary.

   4. Explore peer relationships and involvement in group activities.

   5. Discuss with parents how to achieve a balance between adolescent's appropriate desire for independence and need for consistent, fair limits and someone who will *listen* to concerns.

6. Discuss with patient and parents interpersonal relationships with siblings and parents (individual interview, or joint conference with parents if desired by patient).

7. Discuss with parents the adolescent's need for occasional privacy.

8. Discuss with patient concerns about body image and being different (e.g., acne, tallness, fatness, shortness, delayed puberty).

9. Assess and discuss patient's and parents' attitudes toward alcohol, tobacco and drugs. Counsel as appropriate.

D. Sex education. Extent of counseling at a particular visit will depend on patient's maturity, experience, and stage of development. Special visits with teenager for counseling in this area should be scheduled at appropriate times during adolescence.

1. Discuss patient's relationship with opposite sex and his or her concerns.

2. Assess patient's understanding of anatomy and physiology of reproduction.

3. Assess the immediacy of patient's need for contraceptive information and specific management. Discuss with patient the approach to be taken with parents.

4. Discuss with patient the responsibility that both male and female have for sexual activity and contraception.

5. Discuss venereal disease.

6. Discuss patient's and parents' questions.

E. Safety. Encourage the following:

1. Enrollment in driver-education course.

2. Use of seat belts for automobile safety.

3. Development of swimming, water, and boating safety skills. Never swim alone.

4. Safe use of firearms, if these are available.

F. Other topics, based on patient's and parents' concerns.

VII. Follow-up. In 2 years, or sooner as needed.

Seventeen-Year Clinic Visit

I. Provider. Nurse practitioner.

II. History

A. Interval medical history, including complete review of systems.

B. Review and revision of family and social history.

III. Examination

    A. Measurements (record on growth chart):

        1. Weight.

        2. Height.

    B. Complete physical examination.

IV. Procedures*

    A. Immunizations

        1. Review immunization record.

        2. Tetanus-diphtheria toxoid (adult type-Td), if 10 years have elapsed since previous booster.

    B. Blood pressure (normal is less than 140/90 mm Hg in the supine position).

    C. Hearing screening.

    D. Vision screening.

V. Dental care

    A. Examine teeth.

    B. Discuss rationale for avoiding frequent snacks of sugar-containing foods.

    C. Remind patient to brush teeth twice a day and to floss once a day.

    D. Refer if patient was not seen by dental service within the previous year.

VI. Counseling

    A. Nutrition

        1. Review diet. Counsel on importance of basic food groups. Consider family preferences and economic factors.

        2. Emphasize importance of breakfast.

    B. Physical care

        1. Review home management of illnesses occurring since previous visit.

        2. Discuss importance of adequate sleep and regular exercise.

        3. Discuss patient's questions.

    C. Behavior and psychosocial environment

*See Use of the Health Maintenance Flow Sheet, pp. 1–7, for details.

    1. Discuss school adjustment and progress.

    2. Discuss future career and education plans.

    3. Discuss relationship with opposite sex and his or her concerns.

    4. Discuss interpersonal relationship with parents (individual interview, and joint conference with parents if desired by patient).

    5. Assess and discuss patient's attitudes toward alcohol, tobacco, and drugs. Counsel as appropriate.

D. Sex education

    1. Discuss patient's concerns about relationship with opposite sex.

    2. Discuss contraception and responsibility of both male and female.

    3. Discuss venereal disease.

E. Safety. Encourage the following:

    1. Enrollment in driver-education course. If patient is already driving, emphasize the great risk of injury and death associated with poor driving habits. Review the association of alcohol with automobile accidents.

    2. Discuss use of seat belts for automobile safety. Review statistics establishing their value.

    3. Discuss development of swimming, water, and boating safety skills. Emphasize that one should never swim alone.

F. Other topics, based on patient's concerns.

VII. Follow-up. In 3 years, or sooner if needed. If provider does not care for adults, arrange referral at this visit.

Infant and Child Stimulation Guidelines

Birth to Six Months

I. Language and personal-social development

    A. Talk and sing to the baby even though he cannot understand what you say.

    B. Repeat the noises he makes.

    C. While he is awake, place him where he can see and hear what is going on.

II. Visual, auditory, and tactile stimulation

    A. Hang pictures on the wall or crib where the baby can see them. Cut pictures from magazines or use pictures that older children bring home from school.

B. Hang dangling toys above the baby:

1. Attach ribbon, bright cloth, colored paper, ball, shiny spoon, painted spools, measuring spoons, or rubber jar rings to a string or coat hanger and hang it across the crib.

2. Make a mobile. Cut a circle from cardboard or a plastic bleach bottle. Using thread, tie on colorful cutouts from boxes (e.g., circles, birds, butterflies). Hang the mobile from a light fixture or the ceiling over the crib.

C. Make rattles (noisemakers). Fill small cardboard boxes, plastic salt shakers, or soft drink cans with large stones, bottle caps, poker chips, large buttons, or spools, and tape the end shut. (Use large objects that the baby cannot swallow just in case the rattle comes apart.)

D. Make soft, cuddly toys. Sew two pieces of cloth (old towel, cut in pattern) together and stuff with rags, nylons, cotton batting, facial tissues, or toilet paper, or stuff an old sock or glove.

E. Put the child on a blanket on the floor. Let baby see more of the world around him and have an opportunity to exercise his muscles.

Six to Twelve Months

I. Language and personal-social development

A. Talk to him. Tell him what you are doing to or with him even though he does not understand.

B. Point to objects and people and name them over and over.

C. Play games with him (e.g., patty cake, peek-a-boo, where is Johnny's nose?).

D. Have him in the room with you while he is awake. Let him crawl on the floor and explore, or put him in a walker.

E. Let him see himself in the mirror. Talk to him while he is looking in the mirror—"Look at baby's nose," "Here is Johnny's mouth."

II. Visual, auditory, and tactile stimulation

A. Provide soft, cuddly toys.

B. Make noisemakers:

1. Make a drum out of an empty oatmeal box and give the child a stick with which to bang on it.

2. Fill containers of different shapes with previously mentioned articles (see Birth to Six Months, **II.C**).

C. **Give him objects to handle and explore** (objects that are unbreakable and too large to be swallowed). When the child is in his walker, tie these objects to the walker so that he can handle and play with them.

    1. Let him play with a rolling pin, large spoons, boxes (cereal, shoe, berry, match), bowls, pots, pans, cans, baking tins (cake, pie, muffin), plastic cups, screw-top plastic bottles, coffee pot, bandage cans.

    2. Present a variety of textures (hard, soft, fuzzy, smooth), sponges, different types of material (velvet, imitation fur, cotton, wool) by making a ball out of different textured materials and stuffing it with cotton, rags, or nylons.

D. **Provide fill and dump toys.** Use a container with a large opening (e.g., milk carton, coffee can, oatmeal box) and gather small objects to place in the container and dump out (e.g., spools, measuring spoons, clothespins, corks, poker chips).

E. **Put baby's favorite toy in a paper bag** and have him find it.

One to Three Years

I. **Language development**

A. **Talk to the child.** Listen with interest to what he has to say. Use complete thoughts—not "Pick it up," but "Pick up the ball from under the table."

B. **Read to him** or tell him stories.

C. **Have him tell you stories** about pictures in books or magazines.

D. **Make a picture book.** Cut out large pieces of paper bag for the cover and pages. Fold them in half and tie them together with string or yarn. Paste pictures in the book from magazines, cereal boxes, or newspapers.

E. **Name parts of his body** and pictures of people. Have him name objects.

F. **Let him look in a mirror** and point out his facial features and body parts.

G. **Play singing games** (e.g., "Ring Around the Rosy," "Row, Row, Row Your Boat").

H. **Play telephone** with him.

I. **Play with puppets;** have a conversation using puppets.

    1. Paper bag puppets. Fill the end of a small bag with cotton or crumpled newspaper; insert a stick or pencil; tie a string around the stuffed area; and stick-paint, draw, or color a face on the bag.

2. **Potato puppets.** Insert a stick in a small potato. Create facial features by painting the surface of the potato or using bits of paper held in place with pins.

3. **Potato finger puppets.** Make by cutting a small hole in the bottom of the potato and slipping the potato over one's finger.

4. **Old-glove puppets.** Cut off the fingers and thumb of a glove and stuff them with cotton, nylons, or old rags. The thumb becomes the head and body of the puppet, and two fingers become the arms when sewn to the thumb section. Bind the head and waist sections off with string or yarn. Decorate with pieces of material, yarn, and ribbon.

II. Personal-social development

A. Let the child play with **dolls and stuffed animals.**

B. **Take him on trips** to the store, to a neighbor's house, riding in car or on the bus, to the park and zoo. Point to and name people, objects, and animals.

C. **Play games** such as hide and seek with him.

D. Allow the child to experiment with dressing up and with **adult role playing.**

1. Give the child mother's or father's old hats, dresses, suits, shoes, purses, and wallets.

2. Make hats and masks out of paper bags or paper plates. Make dresses out of blankets or material.

3. Let the child use cooking utensils, house-cleaning equipment, and safe tools.

4. Make a house by putting a blanket over a high table.

III. Gross motor development

A. **Push-pull toys**

1. Attach a string to a large box and fill it with light-weight objects.

2. Make a train by tying boxes (shoe boxes, milk cartons, salt boxes) together with heavy string and attaching a pull string.

B. **Cardboard tunnel to crawl through.** Cut ends off large cardboard boxes and attach several boxes together to make a tunnel.

C. **Climbing stairs**

D. **Walking board.** Rest a board 1 foot wide by 3 feet long on bricks. Encourage the child to walk forward, backward, sideways, and jump down. As the child's coordination improves, decrease the width of the board.

E. **Throwing and catching a ball or bean bag.** Make a large ball out of two pieces of cloth sewn together and stuffed with rags, cotton, or nylons.

F. **Sand play** (using unbreakable things)

1. Use an inner tube as an outside frame for a sandbox and fill the inside area with sand.

2. Give the child spoons, cans, bowls, cups, sieves, and funnels to fill and dump.

3. Cut a bleach bottle in half. Use bottom for a pail (make a handle out of heavy string); use the top for a funnel.

G. **Water play,** outdoors in a large tub or indoors in the sink or bathtub. Give the child unbreakable containers, sponges, cork, bar of soap.

H. **Riding a tricycle**

IV. **Fine motor development**

A. **Fill-and-dump-toys.** As the child's coordination improves, decrease the size of the container and the opening (e.g., plastic milk bottle, small jars and cans) and give him smaller objects to put into the container (e.g., buttons, bottle caps, peas, beans, macaroni).

B. **Sorting activity.** Give the child three containers and bottle caps, buttons, and beans; have him put all the caps in one container, buttons in another, and beans in the other. Later, use the sections of an egg carton.

C. **Stacking toys.** Build a pyramid with different-sized boxes or cans, the largest on the bottom and the smallest on top.

D. **Nesting toys.** Use graduated-sized boxes, bowls, pots, pans, or cups that fit inside one another. Start by using three sizes.

E. **Clothespins and a coffee can or loaf pan.** Have the child put the clothespins on the edge of the can. This can also be used as a sorting activity; paint the pins different colors and have child sort them by color.

F. **Blocks.** Make different-sized blocks from boxes and wood scraps. Cut off the tops of two thoroughly washed milk or cream cartons and push them together. Show the child how to build. Have him copy what you build.

G. **Stringing objects.** Use old shoelaces or heavy string and spools of different sizes. As coordination improves, give the child smaller objects (macaroni and beads).

H. **Puzzles.** Make your own by pasting pictures from magazines onto cardboard and cutting it into pieces. Start with simple pictures of one object and cut into three to five large pieces. With an older child, use a more complex picture and five to ten small pieces.

I. **Large pencil or crayon.** Have the child copy a line or simple shape you make. Allow him to draw whatever he wishes. Use this time to start teaching colors. Use paper bags or cut-up cardboard boxes to draw on.

Three to Five Years

I. **Language development**

A. **Talk to the child,** using complete thoughts and ideas. Listen to him. Encourage him to tell you what he did during the day by asking questions.

B. **Read to him** or tell him stories.

C. **Play singing games** (e.g., "Here We Go Round the Mulberry Bush," "This Is the Way We Wash Our Clothes").

D. **Encourage him to make up stories** about pictures in books and magazines ("Once upon a time . . . ").

E. **Play with puppets.**

II. **Personal-social development**

A. Show him how to **dress himself.**

B. Give him **small tasks** to do around the house (e.g., set table, help clear table, sweep floor, pick up toys).

C. Allow him to experiment with dressing up and **adult role playing.**

1. Let him use old clothes, cooking utensils, house-cleaning equipment, and safe tools.

2. Put chairs together to play train or bus.

3. Make a house under a table.

4. Use paper plates decorated with colored paper, ribbon, or paint to make hats.

5. Use paper bags to make hats and masks.

D. **Grow plants in cans.**

E. Encourage him to play **outdoor games with peers** (e.g., red rover, hide and seek).

III. **Gross motor development**

A. **Cardboard tunnel**

B. **Walking board.** Use a board about 4 inches wide.

C. **Sand play.** Encourage child to build creatively (e.g., make cities).

D. **Water play.** Let child enjoy washing dishes or clothes.

E. Throwing, catching, and batting a ball. Use a small rubber or semihard ball.

F. Throwing a bean bag at a target. Fill an old sock with beans and sew the end shut (reinforce by sewing it several times). Make a target out of a cardboard box folded like an inverted **V** (tent-shaped); attach a heavy string to each side to stabilize it. Cut a hole in one side of the target and paint or color a clown's face around the hole.

G. Rope ladder. Make a ladder out of rope and attach it to a low branch of a tree for the child to climb.

H. Playing jump rope and hopscotch (start between 5 and 6 years of age).

I. Riding a tricycle and bicycle

IV. Fine motor development

A. Fill-and-dump toys.

B. Stacking toys. Increase the number and use smaller objects to be stacked (e.g., spools).

C. Nesting toys. Increase the number and sizes of objects to be nested.

D. Sorting activity. Give the child many objects and ask him to sort them according to color, shape, or function. For example, give the child an egg carton or small cans and colored buttons and have him sort according to color.

E. Blocks. Give him blocks of different sizes and encourage him to build more complicated structures (e.g., houses, farms, forts).

F. Stringing objects. String macaroni or straws cut into small pieces. Make necklaces and bracelets and paint them bright colors.

G. Puzzles. Make more complicated puzzles, using detailed pictures cut into eight to twenty pieces.

H. Pencils and crayons. Use paper bags or cut-up cardboard boxes to draw on. Draw a simple picture and have him color it. Draw simple forms (circles, squares, cross) and have the child copy them. Encourage the child to draw his own pictures.

I. Finger painting

1. Use the want-ad section of newspaper (because it has small, all-over print) or shelf paper for painting paper.

2. Old shirts or blouses make good smocks.

3. Recipe for paint

   1½ cups laundry starch
   1 quart boiling water
   1½ cups soap flakes

Few drops food coloring
½ cup talcum powder (optional)

Mix starch with enough cold water to make a paste, add boiling water, and stir until clear and glossy. Add talcum. Cool mixture. Add soap flakes, and stir until evenly distributed. Mixture should be thick. Add a few drops of food coloring. Pour into jar and cover. Store in a cool place.

J. Clay or play dough

1. Show the child how to make objects and animals.

2. Recipe for play dough

   1 part flour
   1 part salt
   1 part water

   Mix together to a soft consistency. Will keep 3–4 days if wrapped in wax paper and stored in the refrigerator.

K. Collages

1. Paste bits of styrofoam, cotton, cloth, colorful yarn, ribbon, paper, calendars, catalogues, magazines, or pipe cleaners to a piece of cardboard to create a picture. Hang in a place for people to admire.

2. Paste recipe: To a handful of flour add water, a little at a time, until mixture is gooey (should be quite thick so it will not run all over the page). Add a pinch of salt.

L. Sewing cards. Draw a design or picture on a piece of cardboard. Punch holes along the line. Give the child an old shoelace or large needle and yarn to sew with, along the outline.

M. Child's blunt scissors

1. Show child how to hold and use scissors.

2. Give him a long strip of paper ¾-inch wide marked with thick lines at 1-inch intervals. Have him cut off sections with one snip.

3. When he is older give him wider strips sectioned off in large pieces that require several strokes of the scissors.

4. Have the child practice cutting curves. When this is mastered, he can cut circles and other objects.

5. Have him cut zig-zag strips, which become crowns, mountains, Christmas trees.

6. Draw large, simple geometric shapes and have him cut them out.

N. Materials for construction. Give the child wood scraps and nails and help him build things.

Periodic Health Screening: Adult

I. Value of periodic health assessment. The value of periodic screening and examination of well patients remains controversial. Few maneuvers fulfill the criteria of a useful screening procedure: (a) The disease sought is an important problem for which there is a treatment. (b) There is a latent or early symptomatic period during which a screening test is effective. (c) The screening test is available at a reasonable cost and has adequate specificity and sensitivity.

Nonetheless, it has been the experience of most programs that a periodic meeting between patient and health care provider is beneficial. In keeping with this conclusion, we recommend an age-related assessment that includes the most widely recognized screening procedures plus maneuvers that are accepted because they provide baseline information. Nurse practitioners at North Carolina Memorial Hospital have designed a health maintenance flow sheet for use in the medical clinics (Figure 1-2). This flow sheet reflects current thinking about screening procedures; that is, about physical examination and laboratory tests. It did not, however, include health education and inquiry about health habits. The screening physical examination is a poor method of finding disease; the health screening guidelines advocate a directed physical examination that is age and sex related. Part of patient education is to demonstrate that the preventive measures outlined below are an improvement over listening to the heart every year. Preventive health services may be administered during a visit for an acute problem. We (the editors) have adopted the flow sheet and have added questions to explore health habits and needs for counseling.

A. The appropriate frequency of Papanicolaou or Pap smears for detection of cervical cancer remains controversial. The intervals suggested in Figure 1-2 are based on the guidelines published by the American Cancer Society.* Many physicians believe, however, that these recommendations are inadequate and advocate annual Papanicolaou smears. The American Cancer Society recommends that in asymptomatic females over 35 years old, Pap smears may be done once every 3 years following two negative annual smears. Those females at high risk (early age of first intercourse, multiple sexual partners, or other risk factors) may need more frequent examinations. Those with inactive sexual life may need less frequent testing.

B. Routine primary polio vaccination is not recommended for those 18 years old and over residing in the United States. Immunization is recommended, though, for certain adults at greater risk.†

C. Influenza vaccine is recommended** annually for individuals at in-

*Ca-A *Cancer Journal for Clinicians* 30 (No. 28, July/August): 215, 1980.
†MMWR, HEW Publication No. (CDC) 80–8017, Vol. 28 No. 43. Nov. 2, 1979. Pp. 517–518.
**MMWR, HHS Publication No. (CDC) 85–8017, Vol. 35, No. 20, May 23, 1986. Pp. 319–332.

Date												
Age	17	18	19	20	21	22	23	24	25	26	27	28	29
Blood pressure	x	x	x	x	x	x	x	x	x	x	x	x	x
Oral examination				x					x				
Breast/testicles examination	x	x	x	x	x	x	x	x	x	x	x	x	x
Rectal examination													
Stool occult blood													
Pap smear (I.A.)	x	x	x	x	x	x	x	x	x	x	x	x	x
PPD									x				
VDRL									x				
CBC				x					x				
Serum creatinine				x					x				
Urine protein		x		x		x		x		x		x	
Urine sugar		x		x		x		x		x		x	
Diphtheria-tetanus toxoid (I.E.)									x				
Polio vaccine (I.B.)													
Rubella titer (I.F.)									x				
ECG													
Health education (every assessment)													
Nutritional													
Physical care													
Behavior/psychosocial													
Safety (seat belt)													
Sex													
Tobacco/alcohol													

Figure 1-2. Health maintenance flow sheet (adult).

30	31	32	33	34	35	36	37	38	39	40	41	42	43	44	45	46	47	48	49
x	x	x	x	x	x	x	x	x	x	x	x	x	x	x	x	x	x	x	x
x					x					x		x		x		x		x	
x	x	x	x	x	x	x	x	x	x	x	x	x	x	x	x	x	x	x	x
										x		x		x	x	x	x	x	x
										x		x		x	x	x	x	x	x
x	x	x	x	x	x	x			x			x			x			x	
					x										x				
					x										x				
x					x					x					x				
x					x					x					x				
x		x		x		x		x		x		x		x		x		x	
x		x		x		x		x		x		x		x		x		x	
					x										x				
Mammography (Baseline Age 35–40)										x		x		x		x		x	
															x				

| Date | | | | | | | | | | | | | |
Age	50	51	52	53	54	55	56	57	58	59	60	61	62
Blood pressure	x	x	x	x	x	x	x	x	x	x	x	x	x
Oral Examination	x		x		x		x		x		x		x
Breast/testicles examination	x	x	x	x	x	x	x	x	x	x	x	x	x
Rectal examination	x	x	x	x	x	x	x	x	x	x	x	x	x
Stool occult blood	x	x	x	x	x	x	x	x	x	x	x	x	x
Pap smear (I.A.)		x			x			x			x		
PPD						x							
VDRL						x							
CBC	x					x					x		
Serum creatinine	x					x					x		
Urine protein	x		x		x		x		x		x		x
Urine sugar	x		x		x		x		x		x		x
Diphtheria-tetanus toxoid						x							
Influenza vaccine (I.C.)													
Pneumococcal vaccine (I.D.)													
Mammography	x	x	x	x	x	x	x	x	x	x	x	x	x
ECG													
Health education (every assessment)													
Nutritional													
Physical care													
Behavior/psychosocial													
Safety (seat belt)													
Sex													
Tobacco/alcohol													

Figure 1-2 (Continued)

63	64	65	66	67	68	69	70	71	72	73	74	75	76	77	78	79	80	81	82	83	84	85
x	x	x	x	x	x	x	x	x	x	x	x	x	x	x	x	x	x	x	x	x	x	x
	x		x		x		x		x		x		x		x		x		x		x	
x	x	x	x	x	x	x	x	x	x	x	x	x	x	x	x	x	x	x	x	x	x	x
x	x	x	x	x	x	x	x	x	x	x	x	x	x	x	x	x	x	x	x	x	x	x
x	x	x	x	x	x	x	x	x	x	x	x	x	x	x	x	x	x	x	x	x	x	x
x			x			x																
		x										x										x
		x										x										x
		x				x						x					x					x
		x				x						x					x					x
	x		x		x		x		x		x		x		x		x		x		x	
	x		x		x		x		x		x		x		x		x		x		x	
		x										x										x
	x	x	x	x	x	x	x	x	x	x	x	x	x	x	x	x	x	x	x	x	x	x
x	x	x	x	x	x	x	x	x	x	x	x	x	x	x	x	x	x	x	x	x	x	x

creased risk of adverse consequences from infections of the lower respiratory tract. Conditions predisposing to such risk include:

1. **Groups at greatest risk:**
   a. Adults and children with chronic disorders of the cardiovascular or pulmonary systems that require regular medical follow-up or hospitalization during the previous year.
   b. Residents of nursing homes and other chronic care facilities.

2. Groups at moderate risk:
   a. Otherwise healthy persons 65 years of age or older
   b. Adults and children with chronic metabolic disease (including diabetes mellitus), renal dysfunction, anemia, immunosuppression, or asthma requiring regular follow-up or hospitalization in the past year.
   c. Children on long-term aspirin treatment who may be at risk for Reye syndrome.

3. Groups potentially capable of nosocomial transmission to high-risk persons:
   a. Medical personnel
   b. Providers of care to high-risk people in the home setting (family members, visiting nurses, volunteer workers).

D. Pneumococcal vaccine* contains capsular polysaccharides from the 23 most commonly encountered types of pneumococci, replacing the 14-valent vaccine. Patients who have previously received the 14-valent vaccine should not be revaccinated with the 23-valent vaccine and booster shots are not advised. Immunization is recommended for all individuals over 65 years old, and for anyone with increased risk for pneumococcal disease or its complication. The latter group includes:

1. Adults with chronic illnesses, especially cardiovascular disease and chronic pulmonary disease, who sustain increased morbidity with respiratory infections.

2. Adults with chronic illnesses specifically associated with an increased risk for pneumococcal disease or its complications. These include splenic dysfunction or anatomic asplenia, Hodgkin's disease, multiple myeloma, cirrhosis, alcoholism, renal failure, CSF leaks, and conditions associated with immunosuppression.

E. All adults should have a primary series of immunization with tetanus and diphtheria completed and booster given every 10 years.

F. Measles, mumps, rubella—

*MMWR, HHS Publication No. (CDC) 84–8017, Vol. 33, No. 20, May 5, 1986. P. 215.

For measles and mumps, history of disease or immunization record should be sufficient.

For rubella, laboratory evidence of immunity or record of immunization is required.

1. Susceptible adults should be immunized against these diseases; see Chapter 16 for guidelines.

Prostate Cancer Screening

I. Definition. Cancer of the prostate occurs with increasing frequency in males over 50 years of age; only 1 percent of cases occur in males under 50. The cancer usually begins peripherally, grows centrally, and progresses from microscopic disease, to nodule, to local extension, to distant metastasis—bone most frequently. Local lymph nodes also frequently involved.

II. Clinical features

A. Symptoms

1. Most often none until cancer has progressed beyond the prostatic capsule.

2. Occasionally gross or microscopic hematuria.

3. Bone pain from bony metastases.

4. Symptoms of bladder outlet obstruction or irritability are not common unless BPH is also present.

B. Signs

1. Classically a hard nodule in the lateral area of the prostate; larger prostatic masses with obliteration of usual prostatic anatomy not infrequent.

2. With bony metastases, bony tenderness to palpation may be present.

III. Laboratory studies. Acid phosphatase if prostatic cancer is suspected.

IV. Differential diagnosis

A. BPH.

B. Benign adenoma.

C. Prostatic calculus.

V. Screening. Rectal examination and palpation of the prostate remains the most cost-effective and efficient method for detecting prostatic carcinoma. No other method has proven to be better. The correct periodicity for examinations has not been established, but most sources suggest annual examinations in males over 50 years of age. Areas of thickening and induration as well as discrete nodules should be regarded as suspicious.

A. Annual rectal examination in male over 50 with size and consistency of prostate recorded in chart.

B. Stool guaiac may be obtained at the same time.

VI. Consultation-referral. All patients with suspicious areas of induration or a discrete nodule.

Emergencies

2

Anaphylaxis: Pediatric and Adult

I. **Definition.** A hypersensitivity reaction usually occurring within seconds to minutes after exposure to an antigen. The reaction ranges from mild, self-limited symptoms to rapid death.

II. **Etiology.** Agents commonly associated with anaphylaxis include the following. This list is not exhaustive.

   A. **Antibiotics** (especially penicillin and its semisynthetic derivatives).

   B. **Biologicals** (nonhuman sera, gamma globulin, vaccines).

   C. **Local anesthetics.**

   D. **Aspirin.**

   E. **Hymenoptera stings** (bee, yellow jacket, wasp, and hornet).

   F. **Allergic extracts** (skin-testing and treatment solutions).

   G. **Foods** (especially eggs, nuts, and shellfish).

   H. **Intravenous narcotics** (heroin).

   Note: Generally, agents administered parenterally are more likely to result in life-threatening or fatal anaphylactic reactions than those ingested orally or administered topically to mucous membranes. Medications administered orally, such as aspirin or penicillin, however, have been associated with fatal reactions.

III. **Clinical features.** Anaphylaxis is usually characterized by some or all of the following sequence of signs and symptoms. The sooner symptoms develop after the initiating stimulus, the more intense the reaction.

   A. Generalized flush.

   B. Urticaria.

   C. Paroxysmal coughing.

   D. Severe anxiety.

    E. Dyspnea.

    F. Wheezing.

    G. Orthopnea.

    H. Vomiting.

    I. Cyanosis.

    J. Shock.

IV. Laboratory studies. None.

V. Differential diagnosis. The development of symptoms and signs within minutes after contact with an antigen, especially a parenterally administered antigen, makes the diagnosis of anaphylaxis almost certain. An anxiety reaction to an injection might produce some of the symptoms, but consideration of that diagnosis should not result in more than momentary delay in instituting treatment for anaphylaxis.

VI. Treatment

    A. Prevention

        1. Before administering or prescribing any medication, inquire carefully for a history of reactions.

        Note: Anaphylactoid reactions can occur without prior sensitization.

        2. Minimize the use of biologic products (e.g., horse antiserum, unnecessary boosters of tetanus toxoid).

        3. After receiving an agent capable of inducing anaphylaxis (e.g., injection of penicillin, allergy vaccine), the patient should be required to remain in the clinic for at least 15 minutes.

        4. If a patient is allergic to insect venom, he should be counseled to wear a medical alert bracelet; not to go barefoot; to avoid fields of flowers, ripe fruit, bright-colored clothing, and perfume during warm weather; and to carry a kit containing epinephrine and a syringe for injection.

    B. Immediate treatment. Symptoms beginning within 15 minutes after administration of the inciting agent require the most expedient management.

        1. Tourniquet. If an injection has been given into an extremity, a tourniquet should immediately be applied proximal to the site to obstruct venous return from the injection.

        2. Aqueous epinephrine 1:1000

            a. Pediatric dose. 0.01 ml per kg (0.005 ml per lb); maximum single dose, 0.3 ml.

    b. Adult dose. 0.3–0.5 ml.

    c. Inject dose (**a** or **b**) subcutaneously into the upper arm and massage area. Repeat same dose in 5 minutes if necessary.

    d. Also inject same dose (**a** or **b**) one time below the tourniquet around the site of the offending injection or sting to decrease absorption of antigen.

3. Aqueous epinephrine 1:10,000 (1 ml of 1:1000 diluted with 9 ml of IV fluid) should be given intravenously *if patient is in shock.*

    a. Pediatric dose. 0.1 ml per kg (0.05 ml per lb); maximum dose, 3 ml.

    b. Adult dose. 3–5 ml.

4. Airway. Maintain airway and administer oxygen by mask. Hypoxia can result from hypotension and upper airway edema.

5. Intravenous therapy. Start an intravenous infusion and be prepared to administer the following supportive therapy if patient fails to respond to initial therapy or is in shock when first seen. *Steps 1–4 above should always be done first.*

    a. Shock. Give intravenous fluid (normal saline solution *or* lactated Ringer's solution) *rapidly* to support blood pressure. In anaphylaxis, shock results from vasodilation and subsequent inadequate plasma volume.

        (1) Pediatric dose. 20 ml per kg (10 ml per lb) over 15–30 minutes, then slow to 10 ml per kg (5 ml per lb) per hour.

        (2) Adult dose. 1000 ml per 15–30 minutes.

    b. Bronchospasm. Give aminophylline solution intravenously *after shock is controlled.*

        (1) Pediatric and adult dose. 6 mg per kg (3 mg per lb) diluted in 100–200 ml of IV fluid over 10–20 minutes; maximum dose, 500 mg. Inject slowly, not more rapidly than 25 mg/min.

        (2) Reduce dose of aminophylline if patient has received recent theophylline therapy.

6. Record. Maintain a flow sheet with time, vital signs, and medications administered.

7. Consultation. Contact physician for further therapeutic guidance, but do not leave the patient alone.

VII. Complications

    A. Upper airway obstruction. Pharyngeal, uvular, or laryngeal edema, or any combination of these, can develop acutely, especially in children. Observe pharynx frequently. Be prepared to insert oral or endotracheal airway.

B. Lower airway obstruction. Bronchospasm in children may be so severe that decreased tidal volume makes wheezing inaudible.

C. Hypotension. Frequent pulse and blood pressure determinations should be done.

D. Cardiac arrhythmias. Arrhythmias may arise owing to hypoxia, especially in adults.

E. Aspiration of gastric contents. In children, vomiting often accompanies anaphylaxis.

F. Hypoxic seizures

G. Cardiac arrest

VIII. **Consultation-referral.** After instituting immediate therapy **(VI.B)**, contact physician for further therapy and disposition.

IX. **Follow-up**

A. An allergy label should be placed on the front cover of the patient's medical record.

B. If the reaction was to an insect sting, the patient should be referred for desensitization. Follow-up should be done to ensure that desensitization is instituted and that preventive measures **(VI.A.4)** are being taken.

Animal Bites: Pediatric and Adult

I. **Definition and etiology.** Bites of any animal, provoked or unprovoked, excluding snakes (see Snake Bites [Pediatric and Adult]).

II. **Clinical features**

A. Symptoms. Few, other than pain at site of bite.

B. Signs. Puncture wounds or lacerations.

III. **Laboratory studies.** Culture of infected bites.

IV. **Differential diagnosis.** The chief concern is the possibility of rabies in the offending animal. Unprovoked bites must be treated with more suspicion than bites from teased or taunted animals. Bites from wild animals should be treated as rabid unless the animal is found to be free of rabies.

A. Any mammal may carry rabies.

B. The dog is no longer the chief carrier in the United States; other animals, such as skunks, foxes, raccoons, and bats now account for almost 85% of cases of animal rabies annually.

Table 2-1. Summary guide to tetanus prophylaxis in routine wound management: United States, 1985*

History of adsorbed tetanus toxoid (doses)	Clean, minor wounds		All other wounds†	
	Td§	TIG	Td§	TIG
Unknown or < three	Yes	No	Yes	Yes
≥ three¶	No**	No	No††	No

*Important details are in the text.
†Such as, but not limited to, wounds contaminated with dirt, feces, soil, saliva, etc., puncture wounds, avulsions, and wounds resulting from missiles, crushing, burns and frostbite.
§ For children under 7 years old; DTP (DT, if pertussis vaccine is contraindicated) is preferred to tetanus toxoid alone. For persons 7 years old and older, TD is preferred to tetanus toxoid alone.
¶If only three doses of *fluid* toxoid have been received, a fourth dose of toxoid, preferably an adsorbed toxoid, should be given.
**Yes, if more than 10 years since last dose.
††Yes, if more than 5 years since last dose (More frequent boosters are not needed and can accentuate side effects.).

C. Bite: the virus is contained in the saliva of the infected animal and transmitted to the wound by the teeth penetrating the skin; thus, claw scratches do not transmit virus. Nonbite: contamination of open wounds and mucous membranes, or abrasion with saliva from an infected animal.

D. Rabbits, squirrels, chipmunks, rats, and mice are seldom infective.

E. Properly vaccinated animals have only a slight chance of developing the disease.

V. Treatment

A. Wash the wound immediately with copious amounts of soap and water. Then carefully wash away all traces of soap and wash with Zephiran (benzalkonium chloride) solution (Zephiran is inactivated by soap). Alcohol, 40–70%, or povidone-iodine solution may be substituted for Zephiran.

B. Control bleeding.

C. Tetanus prophylaxis in wound management.*

D. Rabies prophylaxis. Consult physician; therapy only after consultation. There appear to be benefits from beginning therapy as soon as possible if a risk of rabies is present. See MMWR, p. 397, Vol. 33, No. 28, July 20, 1984.

*MMWR, HHS Publication No. (CDC) 85–8017 Vol. 34, No. 27, July 12, 1985. P. 422.

VI. Complications

A. Infection at wound site.

B. Rarely, tetanus.

C. Rabies.

VII. Consultation-referral

A. All bites in which there is reasonable suspicion of rabies.

B. All large or dirty bites for instructions, wound management, and rabies and tetanus prophylaxis.

VIII. Follow-up. As recommended by consultant.

Snake Bites: Pediatric and Adult

I. Definition. Snake bites can be classified as those caused by:

A. Nonpoisonous snakes.

B. Poisonous snakes but with no venenation (injection of venom).

C. Poisonous snakes with venenation.

II. Etiology (snakes native to the United States)

A. Pit vipers

1. Varieties

a. Rattlesnakes. Several different rattlesnakes are found in the continental United States with a pattern of distribution such that all areas of the country have one or more species.

b. Copperhead moccasin. This snake is found in southern United States, usually in the highlands.

c. Water, or cottonmouth, moccasin. This snake is found in southern swamps.

2. Description

a. All have **triangular heads.**

b. All have **pits** between each eye and nostril.

c. All have **elliptical** (rather than round) **pupils.**

d. Other features. Rattlesnakes have rattles on the ends of their tails. Water moccasins have white mouths.

3. Severity. Rattlesnake bites generally are more serious than those of other species because of the amount and potency of venom injected by its bite.

B. Eastern coral snake

1. **Location.** Florida, coastal Georgia, and the coastal Carolinas.

2. **Description.** This is a small red and black striped snake with yellow rings separating red from black. Its nose is black, and it does not have a noticeable neck or a spade-shaped or triangular head. It may be confused with the nonpoisonous scarlet king snake, which does not have a black nose.

3. **Severity.** Venom is very toxic and affects the nervous system. Fortunately, the snake is shy and rarely bites.

III. Clinical features of pit viper bites

A. Symptoms (with venenation)

1. Pain at site of bite.

2. Paresthesias of affected part, scalp, tongue, perioral region.

3. General weakness.

4. Faintness and dizziness.

5. Nausea, vomiting, and diarrhea.

Note: Eastern coral snakes cause almost no local symptoms, and systemic symptoms are slow to develop.

B. Signs

1. **General** (if severe venenation)

    a. Hypotension.

    b. Sweating.

    c. Muscle vesiculation.

2. **Local**

    a. Puncture wound.

    b. Swelling and edema.

    c. Erythema.

    d. Ecchymoses.

C. Gradation of wounds

1. **Grade 0** (no venenation). Minimal pain and less than 1 inch of surrounding edema and erythema. *No* systemic involvement. Approximately 20% of pit viper bites produce Grade 0 (no venenation) reactions.

2. **Grade 1** (minimal venenation). Severe pain, and 1–5 inches of surrounding edema and erythema in the first 12 hours after the bite. No systemic involvement.

3. **Grade 2** (moderate venenation). Severe pain and edema, pe-

techiae, and ecchymosis of entire extremity, lymphadenopathy of the affected limb. Sometimes, systemic involvement (e.g., nausea, vomiting, giddiness, shock, and neurotoxic symptoms, such as ptosis, weakness, abnormal reflexes).

4. Grade 3 (severe venenation). Severe pain, edema of entire extremity, and generalized petechiae and ecchymoses. Systemic symptoms appear rapidly.

IV. Laboratory studies. None are necessary before consultation with physician.

V. Differential diagnosis

A. Poisonous versus nonpoisonous snake.

B. Venenation versus nonvenenation. (Pit vipers may not venenate, particularly if the snake has just eaten or struck another object.) Usually symptoms will appear within 10–20 minutes of the bite. If the wound is more than 1 hour old and there is no local edema, pain, or tenderness, then venenation has not occurred.

VI. Treatment

A. All snake bites (including those of nonpoisonous snakes)

1. Clean wound with an antiseptic solution, such as benzalkonium chloride (Zephiran) or povidone-iodine (Betadine), or with soap and water.

2. Carry out tetanus prophylaxis, depending on immunization status (see Animal Bites, Pediatric and Adult, **V.C.**, p. 59).

B. Pit viper bites

1. Bites seen within 1 hour. Administer first aid for all grades of bites seen within 1 hour and suspected of being made by a poisonous snake.

a. Apply a tourniquet above the site of the bite. The tourniquet should be applied just tightly enough to impede lymphatic flow. A different technique for impeding the absorption and spread of the venom consists of placing a firm dressing such as folded gauze or a clean handkerchief over the bite site; with Ace bandage tightly wrap the area of the bite as well as proximal to the bite.

b. Make a single longitudinal incision ⅛–¼ inch in length through the fang marks and about ¼ inch deep or as deep as the fang mark. Apply mechanical suction over the incision for at least 15 minutes.

2. Bites seen after 1 hour. Steps **1a** and **b** are no longer helpful and should not be done.

a. Keep patient quiet and lying down.

b. Do *not* pack extremity in ice or ice water.

c. Do *not* give patient alcohol.

d. Monitor blood pressure, pulse, and respiratory rate every half hour.

e. Be prepared to treat shock.

3. **Specific therapy.** Consult physician for all snake bites. There is good evidence that prompt local excision of the poisonous snake bite wound can remove large amounts of venom and reduce the need for antivenin, particularly for bites by the copperhead. If the decision to give antivenin has been made, first evaluate for sensitivity, and then proceed promptly to administration, because delay decreases the effectiveness.

a. **Evaluating for sensitivity.**
Antivenin (Crotalidae) is in horse serum and can cause immediate anaphylaxis and a delayed serum sickness reaction. Appropriate measures to guard against a severe allergic reaction must be taken:

(1) A careful history of previous allergic reactions or illnesses such as hives, asthma, or drug reaction should be obtained. Specific questions about prior exposure to horse serum and/or allergic reaction to horse serum or horses should be asked.

(2) A skin test should be performed as below prior to the injection of antivenin regardless of the history as obtained above. Inject 0.02–0.03 ml of a 1:10 dilution of antivenin intracutaneously. A control test using Sodium Chloride Injection USP may be used in another site.

If the history for allergy and the skin test are negative, one may proceed with caution to infuse the antivenin IV. If the history and skin test are positive, one must carefully weigh the presumed need for antivenin vs. the likelihood of a severe, perhaps fatal anaphylactic reaction. Techniques for dealing with allergic patients are included in the package insert and in the PDR. A syringe of aqueous epinephrine (1:1000 dilution) should be readily available at all times when using antivenin in case of severe allergic reaction.

b. **Dosage and route of administration.** Antivenin should be given by IV drip. To administer, prepare a 1:1 to 1:10 dilution of the reconstituted antivenin in Sodium Chloride for injection USP or 5% Dextrose Injection USP.

(1) **Grade 0.** No antivenin.

(2) **Grade 1.** 2–4 vials (20–40 ml) antivenin (Crotalidae) poly-valent* IV.

(3) **Grade 2.** 5–9 vials (50–90 ml) antivenin IV. Do sensitivity test first (see **a**).

(4) **Grade 3.** 10–15 vials (100–150 ml) antivenin IV. Do sensitivity test first (see **a**).

C. **Coral snake bites**

1. Any person who is bitten by a coral snake and who has a break in the skin from teeth or fangs should be referred to a physician and observed for 48 hours.

2. If there are fang marks, wash the lesion and apply a tourniquet until consultation can be obtained.

3. Refer to physician and obtain North American coral snake antivenin.*

VII. **Complications**

A. Respiratory depression.

B. Cardiovascular collapse.

C. Coma.

D. Local necrosis.

E. Infection of wound.

F. Joint disability.

G. Loss of digits or extremity.

VIII. **Consultation-referral.** Consult physician for management of all snake bites.

IX. **Follow-up.** All persons receiving antivenin should be told of the possible symptoms of serum sickness (malaise, arthralgia, urticaria, swelling of lymph nodes, fever). Should any of these develop (usually within 8–12 days), patient should return.

Minor Burns: Pediatric and Adult

I. **Definition.** Thermal injuries to the skin, which may be

A. **First degree.** Erythema only.

*Wyeth Laboratories, P.O. Box 8299, Philadelphia, PA 19101.

B. Second degree (partial thickness). Blister formation with or without peeling and weeping.

C. Third degree (full thickness). Early, may have charred or whitish appearance and areas of anesthesia.

II. **Etiology.** Contact with any heat source. The degree of damage depends on the duration of exposure and the source of heat. Scalds generally cause second-degree burns, whereas flame or hot metal may cause third-degree burns.

III. **Clinical features**

   A. Symptoms. Usually only pain. Severe burns with nerve damage may be less painful than first- or second-degree burns.

   B. Signs. See I.

IV. **Laboratory studies.** None.

V. **Differential diagnosis.** Consider abuse or neglect in pediatric age group and in the elderly or mentally retarded.

VI. **Treatment**

   A. First degree burn

   1. Plunge affected area into cold water for several minutes, if less than 45 minutes have elapsed since burn injury.

   2. Clean gently with soap and water.

   3. No dressings are necessary.

   B. Second degree burn

   1. Plunge affected area into cold water for several minutes, if less than 45 minutes have elapsed since burn injury.

   2. Clean gently with soap and water.

   3. Leave blisters intact but may perform simple debridement of open blisters.

   4. Cover burned area with silver sulfadiazine 1% cream (Silvadene) nonadherent gauze, and bulky dry sterile dressing.

   5. Carry out tetanus prophylaxis; see Animal Bites (Pediatric and Adult), **V.C.,** p. 59.

   C. Third degree burn. Refer to physician in all cases.

VII. **Complications.**

   A. Bacterial infection.

   B. Progression of second to third degree, if infection develops.

VIII. **Consultation-referral**

  A. All third-degree burns that totally or partially involve the burned area.

  B. Extensive second-degree burns that involve an area greater than that covered by examiner's hand.

  C. Facial burns.

  D. Any suspicion of child abuse or neglect.

 IX. Follow-up

  A. First degree burn. None.

  B. Second degree burn

   1. Have the patient return in 2 days for dressing change.

   2. Have the patient return every 1–2 days thereafter until epithelialization occurs without infection.

Cardiac Arrest: Pediatric and Adult

 I. Definition. The cessation of effective cardiac function due to either a failure of electrical excitation (cardiac standstill) or an arrhythmia that does not permit effective ventricular contraction (e.g., ventricular fibrillation).

 II. Etiology. Cardiac arrest may be associated with any severe illness, but in an ambulatory setting it usually occurs in persons with acute or chronic cardiac or respiratory disease, that is, arteriosclerotic heart disease with or without myocardial infarction or chronic obstructive pulmonary disease. In children, cardiac arrest is much more likely to be caused by hypoxia (with or without airway obstruction).

 III. Clinical features

  A. Symptoms. Associated with underlying disease.

  B. Signs

   1. Absent pulses and blood pressure. (See also shock, p. 83.)

   2. Unconsciousness.

   3. Absent or gasping respirations.

   4. Cyanosis.

 IV. Laboratory studies. There is no need for laboratory tests other than blood gases and pH during the acute episode surrounding a cardiac arrest.

 V. Differential diagnosis. See II.

 VI. Treatment. Ultimately, treatment depends on etiology; initially, however, there are certain things that must be done once it has been determined that there is no blood pressure and that heartbeat is either absent or irregular and ineffective. If a physician is not present and the patient is a candidate for resuscitation, the nurse practitioner should notify physician and begin the following measures with assistance from other clinical personnel:

A. Call for help and notify physician.

B. Airway measures

1. Examine the airway for foreign objects.

2. Pull jaw forward and tilt neck. A mouthpiece that holds the tongue forward may be useful.

3. Begin mouth-to-mouth resuscitation, or if available use an Ambu bag.

4. Attach oxygen to Ambu bag as soon as it becomes available.

5. Suction secretions present in the mouth and throat frequently.

6. See Table 2-2 for proper rate of ventilation.

7. A nasogastric tube is usually helpful to prevent vomiting.

C. External cardiac massage*

1. If patient is lying on couch or other soft surface, place board under his or her back. If no board is available, quickly transfer patient to floor.

2. Place hands on lower sternum (midsternum in a young child) so that downward pressure will compress the heart between the sternum and the spinal column. For adults arms should be relatively stiff so that pressure is applied from the shoulder through the heels of the hands.

3. Begin cardiac massage with rhythm of 5 heartbeats per breath and rate of 1 beat per second. See table for rate in children.

4. External massage should generate a pulse. Evaluate success by palpating a large artery, such as the femoral or brachial arteries.

D. Place an intravenous line.

1. Use one of the following fluids to keep the IV line open for medication.

   a. 0.9% saline solution

      or

*JAMA, 255: No. 21, 2905–2984, June 6, 1986.

Table 2-2. Suggested ventilation/sternal compression rates in children

	0–18 mos.	18 mos.–6 yr.	6 yr.–10 yr.	Over 10 yr.
Site of Compression	midsternal	midsternal	lower third of sternum	lower third of sternum
Rate of Compression	100/min.	80/min.	70/min.	60/min.
Rate of Ventilation*	20/min.	15/min.	15/min.	12/min.

*This is the minimal rate of ventilation. Hyperventilation is often useful.

      b. 5% dextrose in water

      or

      c. Any available standard IV solution.

   2. Begin flow sheet to record drug administration and vital signs

   3. Sodium Bicarbonate is no longer routinely used and should not be administered at this time.

E. Obtain initial ECG

   1. No electrical activity. Deliver blow to the chest.

   2. Ventricular fibrillation. Begin defibrillation at 2–3 watt-seconds/kg in children, 200 watt-seconds in adults, if the following conditions apply:

      a. No pulse or heartbeat is detectable.

      b. An airway has been established and oxygen therapy begun

      c. A blow to the sternum has not generated a heartbeat.

      d. Ventricular fibrillation is likely or is seen on ECG. If initial defibrillation is ineffective, increase voltage to 300 watt-seconds in adults and double the voltage in children and repeat defibrillation.

F. Treatment without defibrillation. If there is no defibrillator available or no one present trained in its use, maintain assisted respiration and external cardiac massage (see **B** through **D** above).

   1. No electrical activity. Epinephrine 1:10,000, 5 ml in adult, 0.1 ml/kg in children, directly into IV tubing or intracardiac. Repeat every 3–5 minutes as needed to maintain heartbeat.

   2. Electrical activity without palpable pulse (electromechanical dissociation).

      a. Continue CPR.

   b. Epinephrine as above.

   c. Consider Na Bicarbonate, 1 meg/kg, and repeat half original dose every 10 minutes.

3. Ventricular fibrillation. Although in this situation chemical intervention is rarely effective, one may try the following:

   a. Lidocaine, 20 mg per milliliter, 4–5 ml (80–100 mg) directly into IV line over 2–4 minutes (use IV lidocaine labeled for cardiac arrythmias, which has no preservatives.) 1 mg/kg IV bolus for children.

   b. If initial dose of lidocaine does not stop fibrillation, repeat in 10–15 minutes.

   c. Bretylium 5 mg/kg bolus (500 mg in adult). May double dose in 10 minutes.

G. Final steps. Continue resuscitation until heartbeat and adequate respiration are restored. The patient then should be transferred to a hospital as soon as a vehicle with support equipment is available. Discontinue resuscitation after consultation with a physician.

VII. Complications

A. Central nervous system damage from hypoxia.

B. Renal tubular necrosis.

C. Adult Respiratory Distress Syndrome (Shock Lung).

VIII. Consultation-referral. All patients, after lifesaving measures have been initiated.

IX. Follow-up. Varies with each patient.

Convulsions: Pediatric

I. Definition. Tonic or clonic muscular contractions, or both, usually associated with unconsciousness. They are expressions of abnormal electrical discharge of neurons in the central nervous system (CNS).

A. The terms *convulsions, seizures, epilepsy,* and *fits* may be used synonymously by patients.

B. This definition applies to major motor convulsions only. Any unexplained, episodic alteration of consciousness could represent a seizure or abnormal electrical discharge in the CNS.

II. Etiology (list is not exhaustive).

A. Neonatal period

   1. Anoxic CNS injury.

    2. Birth trauma.

    3. CNS infection.

    4. Hypoglycemia.

    5. Hypocalcemia.

    6. Congenital abnormalities of the CNS.

B. Infancy

    1. Febrile convulsions.

    2. CNS infection.

    3. Residual damage from prenatal or perinatal causes.

    4. CNS trauma.

    5. Ingestion of drugs or poisons.

    6. Ischemia or anoxia, such as breath-holding spells.

C. Childhood

    1. Idiopathic and familial epilepsy.

    2. Residual damage from prenatal or perinatal causes.

    3. CNS infection.

    4. Ingestion of drugs or poisons.

    5. CNS trauma.

    6. Glomerulonephritis.

    7. Brain masses.

III. Clinical features (depend to some extent on age and etiology.)

  A. Symptoms

    1. Sometimes, short prodrome of irritability, anorexia, headache, and lethargy.

    2. Symptoms characterizing underlying disorder.

  B. Signs (usual sequential evolution; may be great variation, however, depending in part on underlying disorder).

    1. Usually, abrupt onset of tonic muscular contraction.

    2. Tonic spasm often occurring simultaneously with loss of consciousness.

    3. Facial pallor, often followed by erythema and then cyanosis, depending on length of tonic spasm of respiratory muscles.

    4. Eyeballs rolled upward or to one side.

5. Head hyperextended or turned to one side. Contorted expression caused by contraction of facial muscles.

6. Abdominal and chest muscles in tonic spasm, often accompanied by urination and occasionally by defecation.

7. Clonic phase (rhythmic contraction of muscles), localized or generalized, and lasting for a variable period of time.

8. Often, sleep or lethargy.

IV. **Laboratory studies.** After consultation. Tests depend on suspected underlying cause. (Save blood for glucose determination, or do Dextrostix before giving glucose.)

V. **Differential diagnosis**

   A. Tremulousness associated with high fever or chill, or both.

   B. Hysterical episodes. Hypoglycemia can cause both behavior disturbances and convulsions.

   C. Breath-holding spell causing unconsciousness. Occasionally breath-holding spell can lead to enough anoxia to cause a convulsion.

VI. **Treatment.** In the great majority of cases convulsions are self-limited and cease before treatment is instituted. Occasionally more harm is done by overtreatment than by observation.

   A. **General measures**

   1. Maintain a clear airway by turning the patient on one side with head low to encourage gravity drainage of secretions and vomitus and to prevent aspiration. Suction when necessary.

   2. Give oxygen.

   3. Place the patient in such a position as to prevent injury by falling or knocking against objects.

   4. Do *not* try to pry clenched jaws apart to place an object between teeth.

   5. Observe and be able to describe the duration and focal elements of the convulsion, which include:

      a. Unusual behavior before the convulsion.

      b. Movements of one part or side of the body early or late in the convulsion.

      c. Persistent weakness of one part of the body after the convulsion has occurred.

   B. **Specific therapy**

   1. **History.** Obtain a brief history sufficient to discover any etiologic disorder that will respond to specific therapy, for example:

Table 2-3. Rectal dose of paraldehyde per body weight, as an anticonvulsant

Body weight	Paraldehyde (ml)[a] (0.3 m per kg per dose)
3–5 kg (6–10 lb)	1.2
5–7 kg (10–15 lb)	1.8
7–9 kg (15–20 lb)	2.4
9–11 kg (20–24 lb)	3.0
11–13 kg (24–29 lb)	3.6
13–15 kg (29–33 lb)	4.2
15–17 kg (33–37 lb)	4.8
17–19 kg (37–42 lb)	5.4
Over 19 kg (over 42 lb)	6.0

[a]Mix this dose of paraldehyde with an equal volume of mineral oil and give as a retention enema. Avoid plastic equipment. Measure in a glass syringe. Paraldehyde is contraindicated in hepatic or pulmonary disease.

    a. Insulin-induced hypoglycemia.

    b. Intracranial hemorrhage caused by head trauma.

    c. Hyponatremia from treatment of prolonged diarrhea by non-sodium-containing fluids.

    d. High fever prior to convulsion.

    e. Renal disease suggesting hypertensive encephalopathy.

2. Paraldehyde should be administered *rectally* under the following circumstances:

    a. A convulsion has lasted for more than 10 minutes

    or

    b. Three or more separate convulsions have occurred in the preceding 30 minutes.

3. Transfer of patient. If a physician consultation is not available at the time paraldehyde is given, transfer the patient, accompanied by trained personnel, to a facility where a physician is available.

4. Phenobarbital should be administered intramuscularly (see Table 2-4) under the following circumstances:

    a. A convulsion has not stopped within 30 minutes after rectal administation of paraldehyde

Table 2-4. Intramuscular dose of phenobarbital per body weight, as an anticonvulsant

Weight	Phenobarbital (mg)	Volume (ml) of a 130 mg per ml solution
3–4 kg (7–9 lb)	60	0.45
4–5 kg (9–11 lb)	75	0.60
5–6 kg (11–13 lb)	90	0.70
6–7 kg (13–15 lb)	105	0.80
7–9 kg (15–20 lb)	135	1.00
9–11 kg (20–24 lb)	165	1.25
11–13 kg (24–29 lb)	195	1.50
13–16 kg (29–35 lb)	240	1.85
16–19 kg (35–42 lb)	285	2.20
19–22 kg (42–49 lb)	330	2.55
22–26 kg (49–57 lb)	390	3.00
26–31 kg (57–68 lb)	465	3.60
31–37 kg (68–82 lb)	555	4.25
Over 37 kg (over 82 lb)	585	4.50

or

   b. A second convulsion starts within 30 minutes after rectal administration of paraldehyde

   and

   c. A physician consultation or transfer is still not available.

VII. Complications

   A. Aspiration of vomitus causing pneumonitis or lung abscess.

   B. Prolonged anoxia causing CNS injury.

   C. Traumatic injury during convulsion.

   D. Complications of the underlying disorder.

   E. Cardiorespiratory depression caused by anticonvulsants.

VIII. Consultation-referral. A physician should be consulted concerning all convulsing patients, even if convulsions stop spontaneously before patient arrives in the clinic. Therapy may be started while the consultant is being contacted.

   IX. Follow-up. As recommended by consultant.

Convulsions: Adult

I. **Definition.** Clonic or tonic muscular contractions, or both, usually associated with unconsciousness. Contractions are often accompanied by salivation and followed by incontinence.

II. **Etiology**

  A. **Idiopathic epilepsy**

   1. Initial onset may occur in adulthood but most frequently happens in childhood and puberty.

   2. Seizure in a known epileptic.

  B. **Drug withdrawal** (most commonly, barbiturates)

  C. **Alcohol withdrawal.** Usually short-lived and occurring as one seizure or repeated seizures within a space of a few hours during the first several days after withdrawal.

  D. **Hypoglycemia.** The effects of hypoglycemia on CNS range from inappropriate behavior to confusion to coma.

  E. **Hypertensive encephalopathy**

  F. **Cardiac arrhythmia.** Seizures associated with arrhythmias are usually short-lived and generally have only the tonic component.

  G. **Expanding brain lesion**

III. **Clinical features**

  A. **Symptoms**

   1. History of

    a. Epilepsy.

    b. Use of insulin or oral hypoglycemic agents.

    c. Hypertension.

    d. Alcohol or drug abuse.

    e. Situational problems and emotional stress, particularly in young females.

   2. No obvious cause.

   3. Classic cry at beginning of seizure.

  B. **Signs** (usual sequential evolution: may have great variation, however, depending in part on underlying disorder).

   1. Usually, abrupt onset of tonic muscular contraction.

   2. Tonic spasm often occurring simultaneously with loss of consciousness.

3. Facial pallor, often followed by erythema and then cyanosis, depending on length of tonic spasm of respiratory muscles.

4. Eyeballs rolled upward or to one side.

5. Head hyperextended or turned to one side. Contorted expression caused by contraction of facial muscles.

6. Incontinence, abdominal and chest muscles in tonic spasm, often accompanied by urination and occasionally by defecation.

7. Clonic phase (rhythmic contraction of muscles), localized or generalized, and lasting for a variable period of time.

8. Often, sleep or lethargy.

IV. Laboratory studies. None necessary in the case of an actively convulsing patient.

V. Differential diagnosis

A. See **II.**

B. Occasionally a hysterical patient may mimic movements of a convulsion.

VI. Treatment

A. History of a seizure. Refer to physician for:

1. Diagnosis

   or

2. Regulation of drugs, if seizure was in a known epileptic.

B. Active convulsion. Nurse practitioners should not attempt to treat convulsions alone, unless there is no alternative. The following are guidelines for treating adults until transfer or consultation is obtained. Most seizures are self-limited and may stop during evaluation. Occasionally more harm is done by overtreatment than by observation.

1. **General measures**

   a. Maintain a clear airway by turning the patient on one side with head low to encourage gravity drainage of secretions and vomitus and to prevent aspiration. Suction when necessary.

   b. Give oxygen for cyanosis.

   c. Place patient in such a position as to prevent injury by falling or knocking against objects.

   d. Do *not* try to pry clenched jaws apart to place an object between the teeth.

   e. Observe and be able to describe the duration and focal elements of the convulsion (see Convulsions [Pediatric], **VI.A.5** p. 71).

   f. Monitor respirations, blood pressure, temperature, and pulse.

2. Specific therapy

   a. If after above assessment, patient is still having seizure:

   (1) Start IV infusion.

   (2) Give 20 ml of 50% glucose IV.

   b. If no response in 5 minutes, give up to 10 mg of diazepam (Valium) IV over 3–5 minutes.

   Note: Phenytoin takes sufficiently long for effective therapeutic action that it is not used initially to terminate seizures. Acute initiation of phenytoin therapy requires a loading dose and should *not* be done without physician consultation.

VII. Complications

   A. Status epilepticus.

   B. Aspiration.

   C. Traumatic injury during convulsion.

   D. Complications of underlying disorder.

VIII. **Consultation-referral.** Consult on all seizures, but therapy may be started.

IX. **Follow-up.** Individualize for patient or cause of seizure.

Minor Head Injuries: Pediatric and Adult

   I. Definition. Trauma to the head that does *not* result in any alteration of cerebral function.

   II. Etiology. A blow to the head occurring in any of a host of circumstances in which either an object strikes the skull or the skull strikes an object.

   III. Clinical features. The nurse practitioner should manage *only* those patients having minor head injuries as defined by the following positive and negative symptoms and signs:

   A. Symptoms

   1. *No* loss of consciousness at time of injury.

   2. *No* alteration in sensorium from the time of injury until the patient is seen and evaluated.

   3. *No* nausea or vomiting.

   4. *No* focal neurologic symptoms.

   5. Sometimes, minimally to moderately severe headache.

B. Signs

   1. Normal vital signs.

   2. *No* palpable defect on examination of the skull.

   3. Sometimes, localized area of tenderness over the skull.

   4. *No* discharge from the ears.

   5. *No* discharge from the nose.

   6. *No* blood behind tympanic membranes.

   7. Full consciousness, alertness, and orientation to time, person, and place.

   8. Intact cranial nerves.

   9. *No* weakness on motor testing.

   10. *No* demonstrable sensory loss.

   11. Intact and symmetric reflexes.

   12. Flexor plantar response.

IV. Laboratory and other studies. None indicated in minor head injury.

V. Differential diagnosis. Minor head injury (see **III**) must be differentiated from all other head injuries.

VI. Treatment. Careful observation. The patient *may* be allowed to go home if:

   A. There is a competent person who will assume responsibility for observing the patient carefully.

   B. Detailed written instructions as to the nature of the observations to be made are provided. Figure 2-1 is an example of the type of written instructions to be given to the patient's family.

VII. Complications. Even a minor head injury can result in severe complications, such as subdural or epidural hematoma, and can result in rapid deterioration of the patient's neurologic status and severe disability or death.

VIII. Consultation-referral. All head injuries that do not fit the definition of a minor head injury according to these guidelines.

IX. Follow-up. See **VI** and Figure 2-1.

Observation after Head Injury

The patient should be checked every 2 hours for the first 24 hours after the injury. If he is asleep, he should be awakened. If any of the following signs are noted, please call the nurse practitioner (NP) immediately or return the patient to the clinic as soon as possible.

1. Patient unusually sleepy or hard to wake up.
2. Patient mentally confused. Does not know who he is or where he is. Does not recognize familiar people or places.
3. Patient very restless, disturbed, or agitated. Being upset is normal after an accident, but when a patient becomes very nervous and excited after having been quiet and calm, it is important to report it.
4. Nausea and vomiting (complains of being "sick to my stomach" or is throwing up).
5. Severe headache.
6. Difference in the size of the pupils of the eyes. The pupil is the round, dark part of the center of the eye. Normally, pupils are both the same size.
7. Weakness of the arms or legs. This sign is especially important if it is only on one side of the body.
8. Fits, seizures, or convulsions.
9. Drainage of fluid from the ears or nose.

Guidelines for Care at Home

1. The patient may move around and be up as much as he desires.
2. He may eat or drink anything, except *no* alcoholic beverages.
3. If the patient takes medicines regularly, he should be advised by a physician about taking these medicines after head injury.
4. For mild headache, the patient should lie flat until the headache goes away.

_____

NP or MD

I understand the above instructions:

_____

Signed

_____

Relationship to patient

_____

Date

Figure 2-1. Instructions for home observation of a patient after head injury.

Ingestions and Poisonings: Pediatric

I. Definition

   A. Ingestion or absorption of any nonfoodstuff.

   B. Accidental ingestion of a medicine.

II. Etiology. Almost every substance has probably been ingested by children. Commonly ingested toxic substances include acetaminophen, iron tablets, petroleum products, psychotropic drugs (antidepressants, tranquilizers), and aspirin.

III. Clinical features. Ingestions are most common under 5 years of age.

   A. History

      1. The ingestion is often witnessed, or an empty container is found where the child could have ingested its contents.

      2. Ingestions are more likely to occur during periods of disruption or stress in the household.

      3. Someone in the household may be on drug therapy.

      4. Accidental ingestion or other accidents have occurred in the past.

      5. Child under 1 year of age may be receiving an excessive dose of medication.

      6. Any ingestion in a developmentally normal school-age child may be a suicide attempt, and this possibility should be pursued.

   B. Symptoms and signs

      1. Symptoms and signs are likely to be absent if the ingestion is discovered or suspected soon after it occurred. Many ingested substances have low toxicity and will produce no symptoms or signs.

      2. Poisonings and overdosage of medicines can cause a great variety of symptoms and signs, often simulating natural diseases. Consider poisoning especially under the following circumstances:

         a. History suggests (see **A**).

         b. Patient aged 1–4 years.

         c. Very sudden onset of symptoms.

         d. Abnormal odor to breath or clothes.

         e. Unexplained findings, especially unconsciousness, in any patient.

IV. Laboratory studies. As suggested by consultant. Save vomitus, gastric contents, empty containers, and urine.

V. Differential diagnosis

  A. Nonaccidental ingestion

  1. Suicide attempt in child over 5 years of age.

  2. Child abuse or neglect.

  B. Natural diseases (depending on symptoms and signs).

VI. Treatment

  A. Prevention. Advise parents on the following preventive measures

  1. Label all containers with contents.

  2. Keep medicines in safety-cap containers. Always replace cap after use.

  3. Lock all medicines and poisons away and out of reach of children.

  4. Do not store nondrinkable or nonedible substances in drink or food containers.

  5. Keep syrup of ipecac in the house.

  6. Caution parents about the risks of ingestions during disruptive periods in the household (e.g., moving, house painting, emotionally stressful situations).

  B. Telephone calls about ingestion

  1. Try to determine what and how much was ingested and when it was ingested.

  2. Ask that the remainder of the ingested substance and its container be brought with the patient to the clinic. If uncertain what might have been ingested, have all potentially ingested materials that are available in the household brought with the patient (e.g., medications).

  3. *If no contraindications to vomiting exist* (see **E.2**), vomiting may be induced before leaving home or on the way to the clinic to decrease potential toxicity. Syrup of ipecac should be available in every household as part of health maintenance procedures and may be given by parents to induce vomiting (see **E.1** for dosage).

  C. General supportive therapy (as needed)

  1. **Maintenance of airway**

    a. Suction of secretions.

b. Head turned to side and lower than stomach to avoid aspiration of vomitus.

c. Jaw thrust, head tilt, oral airway.

2. Cardiopulmonary resuscitation

3. Control of convulsions. See Convulsions (Pediatric), **VI,** p. 71.

4. Treatment of shock. Start administering intravenous fluids (normal saline solution or Ringer's solution) in a dose of 20 ml per kilogram of body weight (10 ml per pound) over 15–30 minutes.

D. Consultation. Seek consultation, especially from poison control center, before further therapy if consultant is immediately available.

E. Induction of emesis. If consultant is not immediately available and ingestion is suspected, induce emesis with syrup of ipecac, if not contraindicated. (Do not wait for symptoms to develop.)

1. Dose of syrup of ipecac to induce emesis, if no contraindications are present (see **E.2**).

a. Six months to one year of age. 10 ml (2 teaspoons) followed by at least 4–6 ounces of clear liquid.

b. Over one year of age. 15 ml (1 tablespoon) followed by at least 6–8 ounces of clear liquid.

Note: If child does not vomit after 20 minutes, the same dose may be repeated once.

2. Contraindications

a. Unconsciousness or diminished level of consciousness

b. Convulsions

c. Ingestion of corrosives (strong alkali or acid), such as toilet bowl cleaners and drain cleaners (lye, Drano, Liquid PlumR, Saniflush). This can be suspected if burns are present on the lips or tongue or in the mouth, or there is pain on swallowing.

d. Ingestion of petroleum products (e.g., kerosene, gasoline, furniture polish, cleaning fluid, paint thinner). May be suspected by odor on the breath or clothes or by odor of the container. This is a relative, not absolute, contraindication. For example, a petroleum product may be the solvent for an extremely toxic substance. Contact the poison control center for further guidance.

VII. **Complications.** These vary depending on the substance and amoun
to which the patient was exposed.

VIII. **Consultation-referral.** All patients with established or suspected
ingestion or poisoning.

IX. **Follow-up.** As suggested by consultant.

Overdose of Sedative, Hypnotic, or Opiate Drugs: Adult

I. **Definition.** Alterations in the sensorium usually progressing to coma
as a result of the accidental or intentional ingestion or injection of
large quantities of any one of various central nervous system depres
sants.

II. **Etiology.** Barbiturates, opiates, phenothiazine tranquilizers, and sim
ilar agents. The agent may be taken intentionally in a suicide attempt
or accidentally, as in the injection of an unusually potent "street"
drug, such as heroin.

III. **Clinical features**

A. **Symptoms**

1. Alteration of consciousness is present and usually progresses
rapidly to coma.

2. Respiratory depression is common, including progression to ap
nea.

3. A history obtained from those who bring the patient to the clinic
often is essential in establishing the diagnosis. It is often help
ful to have the patient's pill bottles or other drug containers
brought to the clinic.

B. **Signs**

1. Varying levels of coma are present.

2. Pupils often pinpoint in opiate overdose.

3. Needle tracks may be present on arms at sites of previous IV
injections of heroin.

4. Spontaneous respirations often are absent.

IV. **Laboratory studies.** None indicated in acute situation.

V. **Differential diagnosis**

A. **Trauma**

B. **Cerebrovascular disease** (including all forms of strokes)

C. **Severe metabolic derangements** (including diabetic ketoacidosis
hypoglycemia, and severe uremia)

VI. Treatment

A. Clear and maintain open airway.

B. Maintain respirations. Assisted ventilation by means of mouth-to-mouth respiration or an Ambu bag may be necessary.

C. Start IV infusion of dextrose in water. Give 50 ml of 50% glucose if hypoglycemia is suspected.

D. Carry out gastric lavage if drug ingestion is suspected.

E. Give naloxone HCl (Narcan), 0.4–2 mg, IV if opiate overdose is suggested by the history or physical findings. An initial dose of one mg is frequently used. Additional doses may be administered at 2–3 minute intervals. Most patients with suspected opiate overdose have some response after 2 mg but some patients, particularly those suspected of overdosing with Pentazocine (Talwin), may require more than 2 mg. If no response is observed after 10 mg has been administered, question the diagnosis of narcotic-induced toxicity.

VII. Complications. None in acute situation.

VIII. Consultation-referral

A. Immediate telephone consultation for all patients.

B. Referral as soon as patient is stabilized and adequate help is available (preferably an ambulance or rescue squad).

IX. Follow-up. Close psychiatric management if overdose is a suicide attempt.

Shock: Pediatric and Adult

I. Definition. A clinical state almost always associated with hypotension that leads to inadequate cellular perfusion and is manifested by a clinical syndrome described in III.

II. Etiology.

A. Hypovolemia. Loss of blood or other body fluid (e.g., bleeding, diarrhea, vomiting, and excessive perspiration).

B. Cardiogenic disorders. Myocardial dysfunction includes infarction, arrhythmias.

C. Sepsis. Often from gram-negative organisms.

D. Anaphylaxis

E. Drugs and Toxins. For example, opiates, barbiturates, and hypotensive agents.

F. Heat prostration.

G. **Hypoglycemia**

H. **Hypoxial/asphyxia**

III. **Clinical features**

A. **Symptoms**

1. **General.** Patient manifests anxiousness, dizziness, lightheadedness, confusion, and stupor.

2. **Specific** (related to etiology)

a. **Hypovolemia.** Early in the sequence of events leading to hypovolemic shock, the patient may be syncopal on standing because of orthostatic hypotension. Patient may have a history of severe diarrhea and vomiting or inadequate fluid intake while working outside in hot weather.

b. **Cardiogenic shock.** The characteristic pain of myocardial infarction may predominate and may be accompanied by diaphoresis.

c. **Sepsis**

(1) **Infants.** Poor feeding, lethargy, and fever or hypothermia.

(2) **Older children and adults.** Fever or hypothermia, chills, lethargy, sweating. (Septic shock is seen especially with urinary tract infections in the elderly or in patients with indwelling catheters.)

d. **Anaphylaxis.** Insect sting and drug injection are the most common causes.

e. **Drug.** Patients usually are stuporous or in coma with barbiturate overdose. Hypotensive agents initially cause orthostatic hypotension.

B. **Signs**

1. **General**

a. Hypotension (when shock is from volume depletion, the first manifestation may be orthostatic hypotension).

b. Tachycardia.

c. Cool, moist skin, poor capillary refill.

d. Weak, thready pulse.

e. Sweating.

f. Pallor.

g. Decreased urine output.

2. **Specific** (related to etiology)

   a. **Hypovolemia**

      (1) **Bleeding**

         (a) **External.** Usually obvious, but large quantities of blood may be sequestered in the thigh from fracture of the femur.

         (b) **Internal.** Usually due to trauma or bleeding peptic ulcer manifested by hematemesis or coffee ground vomitus and melena.

      (2) **Dehydration.** Decreased skin turgor, dry mouth, and sunken eyes.

   b. **Cardiogenic shock**

      (1) Findings may be only those cited in **B.1** that are related to lowered cardiac output.

      (2) In severe shock, symptoms of congestive heart failure may be present.

   c. **Sepsis.** Patient usually is febrile, although elderly people, neonates, and patients with gram-negative sepsis may be afebrile or hypothermic. The patient may have signs related to underlying urinary tract infection, meningitis, etc.

   d. **Anaphylaxis**

      (1) **Bronchospasm.** Wheezes, increased expiratory phase are present.

      (2) **Urticaria or angioedema** are sometimes present.

      (3) **Laryngeal edema** (inspiratory stridor)

   e. **Drug.** Patients who have taken enough opiates or barbiturates to cause shock are usually stuporous or in coma.

IV. **Laboratory studies.** Always check blood glucose (BG stick or dextrostix). In the initial assessment of shock there is very little need for most laboratory tests, but if the cause is obscure, hematocrit and blood sugar determinations may be helpful. Do not wait for results before starting treatment. For later blood studies, see **VI.I.**

V. **Differential diagnosis.** See **II.**

VI. **Treatment.** A physician should be consulted about the treatment of all patients. Emergency measures, however, should be started *while* the physician is being contacted.

   A. Call for help from other clinic personnel and notify physician.

   B. Take vital signs. Start a flow sheet and evaluate vital signs every 5 minutes after IV infusion **(F)** has been started.

C. Assess the airway (as in any emergency):

  1. Remove vomitus, if present.

  2. Pull jaw forward.

  3. If laryngospasm is present (upper airway obstruction without foreign body or infection), treat patient as for anaphylactic shock; see Anaphylaxis (Pediatric and Adult), **VI.B,** pp. 56–57).

D. Check breathing (auscultate the chest):

  1. If there are wheezes, consider anaphylaxis (as well as pulmonary edema from heart failure).

  2. Assist ventilation with Ambu bag and mask if necessary.

E. Check cardiac status:

  1. Palpate a major vessel.

  2. Quickly auscultate the heart.

F. Start an IV infusion:

  1. Fluid. Use lactated Ringer's or normal saline solution.

  2. Rate

  a. Adult. Run IV as rapidly as possible up to approximately 20–30 ml per minute in the first 30 minutes (except for cardiogenic shock [see **J.5**]).

  b. Pediatric. See Anaphylaxis (Pediatric and Adult), **VI.B.5.a.(1),** p. 57.

G. Obtain a quick medical history:

  1. Underlying diseases

  a. Heart disease.

  b. Allergy to insect or medication.

  c. Bleeding disorder.

  d. Diabetes mellitus.

  e. Chronic urinary tract infection.

  2. Current history

  a. Insect sting.

  b. Drug injection or ingestion.

  c. Symptoms (vomiting, diarrhea).

  d. Exposure to infection, heat, toxin.

   e. Symptoms of urinary tract infection.

   f. Time course.

H. Do a quick physical examination:

   1. Skin. Petechiae or purpura (occasionally associated with sepsis).

   2. Neck. Rigidity (meningitis).

   3. Chest. Wheezing, rales (anaphylaxis, pneumonia, sepsis).

   4. Heart. Arrhythmias, murmurs.

   5. Abdomen

   a. Size of liver.

   b. Abdominal rigidity (peritonitis).

   c. Flank pain.

   d. Prostatic tenderness.

   e. Stool for occult blood.

   f. Vomitus for blood.

I. Draw blood for:

   1. Glucose.

   2. Blood culture.

   3. Complete blood count differential and platelet count.

   4. Electrolytes.

   5. Blood urea nitrogen.

   6. Future use (hold).

J. Start specific treatment:

   1. Bleeding or hypovolemia. IV fluids have been started, which is initially sufficient and lifesaving until help can be obtained.

   2. Anaphylaxis. See Anaphylaxis (Pediatric and Adult), **VI.B,** pp. 56–57.

   3. Hypoglycemia. 20 ml of 50% dextrose (2 ml/kg of 25% solution for children) should be given IV, without waiting for results of laboratory tests.

   4. Sepsis. IV fluids should be sufficient until help can be obtained.

   5. Cardiogenic shock. If shock and pulmonary edema are present in a setting that suggests myocardial infarction, IV fluid should not be pushed, but an open IV line is essential in administering the drugs necessary to treat this condition after consultation.

VII. Complications

A. Complications of the **etiologic** problem.

B. Complications of shock (generally **end-organ destruction**)

    1. Brain. Ischemia, leaving neurologic deficits.

    2. Kidney. Acute tubular necrosis.

    3. Lungs. Adult Respiratory Distress Syndrome (ARDS, Shock Lung).

VIII. Consultation-referral. All patients require immediate consultation.

IX. Follow-up. Varies with individual patient.

Small Open Wounds: Pediatric and Adult

I. Definition. Lacerations that

A. Are *not* located on the face.

B. Do *not* penetrate the subcutaneous tissue.

C. Are *not* associated with functional disturbance, that is, not involving tendons, ligaments, vessels, or nerves.

D. Have *not* been made by a grossly contaminated object.

E. Are small and sufficiently clean so that the edges can be easily approximated using adhesives or cutaneous sutures. Approximation must be carried out without trimming tissue or placing undue tension on the suture line.

II. Etiology. Any of innumerable objects that could sever the skin.

III. Clinical features. See I.

IV. Laboratory studies. Culture infected wounds.

V. Treatment

A. Wounds that do not require sutures

    1. The primary consideration is to keep the wound clean and dry:

        a. Clean with warm water and soap, making sure that dirt and foreign bodies have been removed.

        b. Cover with a loose bandage that will keep out dirt and protect the wound from trauma.

2. If there is inflammation, the wound should be soaked and washed with soap and water for 15–20 minutes 3–4 times a day, and a clean dressing should be applied at home each day until healing begins; then, daily soaking and dressing are sufficient.

3. Tetanus prophylaxis; see Animal Bites (Pediatric and Adult), **V.C,** p. 59.

B. Wounds that require sutures

1. Do not suture wounds if they are more than 6 hours old, as risk of infection increases with time.

2. Clean the wound with warm water and soap.

3. Irrigate the wound with sterile saline solution.

4. Anesthetize the wound with 1–2% lidocaine (Xylocaine).

5. Palpate or probe the wound for foreign objects, such as glass.

6. Generally, make sutures on the extremities with 4-0 silk or nylon; a larger suture material, such as 2-0 silk, may be used on the soles of the feet.

7. Keep the sutured wound dry and covered with a clean, dry dressing for several days, changing the dressing after the first 24 hours.

8. Remove sutures on the basis of the location of the wound:

   a. Head and trunk (5–7 days).

   b. Extremities (7–10 days).

   c. Soles and palms (10–14 days).

9. Tetanus prophylaxis; see Animal Bites (Pediatric and Adult), **V.C,** p. 59.

VI. Complications

A. Infection.

B. Reopening of the wound.

C. Hematoma in the wound.

VII. Consultation-referral

A. Infected wounds.

B. Fever or chills or other evidence of systemic infection.

C. Facial wounds.

D. Wounds penetrating subcutaneous tissue.

    E. Wounds associated with functional disturbance.

    F. Wounds that cannot be easily cleaned.

    G. Wounds with macerated edges that cannot be easily approximated.

VIII. Follow-up

    A. Return visit for suture removal (see **V.B.8**).

    B. Return visit for complications (describe to patient).

Disorders of the Skin

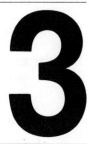

Acne: Pediatric and Adult

I. Definition. Comedones (blackheads, whiteheads), pimples, and tender, red bumps (cysts) on the face, chest, or back, or a combination of these, usually in adolescence or early adulthood.

II. Etiology. Increased activity of sebaceous glands, with obstruction leading to rupture of the glands. Steroids or phenytoin sodium (Dilantin) may produce eruptions in which pustules predominate and comedones are absent.

III. Clinical features

    A. Symptoms

        1. Lesions may be painful.

        2. Stress often can be identified as a precipitating factor.

        3. Psychologic consequences of the condition may be present.

    B. Signs. Increasing numbers of blackheads, whiteheads, pimples, and tender, red bumps on the face, chest, or back are seen, which may lead to pitted scars. One of these lesions may predominate, or all may be present.

IV. Laboratory studies. None.

V. Differential diagnosis

    A. Pyoderma.

    B. Drug eruptions.

VI. Treatment

    A. General measures. Advise patient to do the following:

        1. Keep hands off the face. Avoid picking lesions.

        2. Avoid greasy cleansing creams, oils, and cosmetics.

        3. Shampoo regularly to treat seborrhea, which often accompanies acne.

4. Expect exacerbations even while under treatment, especially during menses and periods of emotional stress.

5. Eat a normal balanced diet. There is *no* need to avoid chocolate or cola.

6. Realize the value of psychological support.

B. Blackheads, whiteheads, papules, and pimples

1. General measures (see **A**).

2. Soaps and astringents.

    a. For very mild acne, wash face with water and any soap 3–4 times a day to remove oil film.

    b. For more extensive acne, use special cleansers (e.g., Fostex) instead of regular soap. Reduce frequency if skin becomes irritated. Discontinue if other topical treatments are used.

3. Drying lotions or gels with benzoyl peroxide 5–10% (Benoxyl, Persadox, Benzagel, Desquam-X) can be applied 1 or 2 times a day. Reduce frequency if excessive dryness or irritation develops.

4. For acne which is predominantly blackheads and whiteheads, tretinoin (Retin A) may be used.

    a. Apply Tretinoin 0.05% cream to dry skin at bedtime. To avoid excessive irritation, begin with use every 2–3 days and increase to daily as tolerated. Caution about sun exposure.

    b. Increase to tretinoin 0.1% cream if necessary, after trial of lower strength for 2 months.

C. Pustules and cysts

1. General measures (see **A**).

2. Soaps and astringents (see **B.2**).

3. Drying lotions (see **B.3**).

4. Topical antibiotic therapy is very effective.

    a. Clindamycin 1% solution (Cleocin T), apply twice daily

    or

    b. Erythromycin 1.5–2% solution (Eryderm, A/T/S, Staticin, T-Stat), apply twice daily.

5. Antibiotic therapy for moderate to severe disease. (To avoid staining baby's teeth, do not use during pregnancy.) Consult physician before starting.

a. Tetracycline, 250 mg 4 times a day, 1 hour before or 2 hours after meals and at bedtime, for 3 weeks. Then decrease to:

b. Tetracycline, 250 mg 2 times a day, 1 hour before or 2 hours after meals, until the lesions are under good control. Then decrease to:

c. Tetracycline, 250 mg daily, for several months.

Note: In some cases tetracycline may be decreased to 250 mg every other day or discontinued completely in the summer. On the other hand, some patients need a continued dosage of 250 mg 2–3 times a day.

d. Tetracycline side effects (*Candida* vaginitis, nausea, vomiting, diarrhea). Patients who do not tolerate tetracycline can be treated with similar doses of erythromycin.

VII. Complications

A. Secondary bacterial infection.

B. Excessive dryness of skin due to overvigorous washing and use of lotion.

C. Tetracycline side effects.

D. Psychologic consequences.

VIII. Consultation-referral

A. Secondary bacterial infection.

B. Resistance to therapy or sudden, persistent worsening after initial improvement.

C. Severe psychologic stress associated with the lesions.

D. Moderate to severe pustular acne requiring antibiotics.

IX. Follow-up

A. Tetracycline treatment

1. Monthly visits until the acne is under good control and the patient is taking a single daily dose.

2. Semi-annual (every 6 months) visits while patient is taking maintenance dose of tetracycline.

B. Nonantibiotic treatment

1. In 2 weeks to assess response.

2. As needed on the basis of the severity of the lesions, the patient's compliance with the regimen, and his or her need for psychologic support.

Atopic Dermatitis: Pediatric and Adult

I. **Definition.** A chronic inflammatory disease of the skin characterized by pruritus and tending to occur in patients with an allergic diathesis. Onset is commonly in infancy after age 2 months.

II. **Etiology.** Unknown. Manifestations are usually secondary to pruritus and scratching of the sensitive skin. The following may initiate and aggravate the itching and inflammation:

   A. Dry skin (cold weather).

   B. Perspiration (hot, humid weather).

   C. Certain foods (orange or tomato juice) on contact with the skin, especially in infants.

   D. Irritating clothing (wool, silk).

   E. Certain soaps, detergents, or cosmetics.

   F. Emotional stress.

III. **Clinical features**

   A. **Symptoms**

   1. Pruritus.

   2. Often, family history of allergic diseases (asthma, allergic rhinitis, urticaria) or atopic dermatitis.

   3. History of asthma and allergic rhinitis (about 50% of cases).

   B. **Signs**

   1. **Infancy**

      a. Rough, erythematous, papular, and occasionally vesicular or scaling eruption, which frequently progresses to weeping and crusting.

      b. Onset after 2 months of age.

      c. Located commonly on cheeks, scalp, postauricular area, neck, and extensor surface of forearms and legs; occasionally on trunk and diaper area.

      d. Fairly rapid alteration between quiescent periods and exacerbations.

      e. Frequent rubbing of involved areas by infant.

      f. In many patients, resolution of the condition by age 2.

   2. **Childhood**

   a. Less weeping and crusting, and more dry, papular, scaling eruption with hypopigmentation.

   b. Intensely pruritic and excoriated lesions.

   c. Located commonly on flexor surfaces of wrists and on antecubital and popliteal areas.

3. **Adolescence and adulthood**

   a. Dry, thickened skin, with accentuation of normal lines and folds; often, hyperpigmentation.

   b. Located commonly on flexor areas of extremities, eyelids, back of neck, and dorsum of hands and feet.

IV. **Laboratory studies.** None.

V. **Differential diagnosis**

   A. Seborrheic dermatitis (sometimes impossible to differentiate in infancy).

   B. Fungal infections of the skin.

   C. Contact dermatitis (e.g., poison ivy).

   D. Irritant dermatitis (e.g., diaper dermatitis).

   E. Rare systemic diseases of infancy associated with an atopic dermatitis type of rash (e.g., phenylketonuria, Wiskott-Aldrich syndrome, histiocytosis X, acrodermatitis enteropathica).

VI. **Treatment**

   A. Patient should avoid factors that initiate pruritus and irritate skin. Advise patient to:

   1. Spend time outdoors in warm weather. Humidify home in winter if heating system dries air.

   2. Prevent dry skin by:

      a. Minimizing duration of soap exposure during bathing. Exposure to water is beneficial. Use a mild soap (e.g., Neutrogena, Tone, Caress, Dove, Touch).

      b. Applying agents that seal water into the skin after it is moistened by a bath or shower (e.g., Alpha-Keri, Domol, Nivea, Aquaphor, Eucerin, petrolatum).

   3. Use warm water for brief baths or showers. Hot water causes pruritus.

   4. Use soft cotton clothing and bedding. Avoid wool, starched, or rough clothing.

Table 3-1. Oral dosage of diphenhydramine HCl (Benadryl) as an antipruritic and sedative

Drug form	Body weight	Dose	Frequency
Benadryl elixir	8–10 kg (18–22 lb)	5.0 ml	
(12.5 mg per 5 ml)[a]	10–15 kg (22–23 lb)	7.5 ml	
	15–20 kg (33–44 lb)	10.0 ml	
	20–30 kg (44–66 lb)	15.0 ml	3 or 4 times a day
or			
Benadryl capsules	15–25 kg (33–55 lb)	1 capsule	
(25 mg per capsule)	Over 25 kg (over 55 lb)	2 capsules	

[a]Caution: May cause drowsiness.

5. Place a cotton pad under the bed sheets to further separate an infant from a plastic mattress.

6. Keep fingernails short.

B. Therapy of active dermatitis:

1. If lesions are weeping or crusted, patient can apply soft cloth compresses of clear water at room temperature for 15 minutes 4 times a day for softening and debridement of crust and control of exudative reactions and pruritus.

2. After an acute, exudative phase has been controlled, patient should apply a corticosteroid to the affected area.

   a. Hydrocortisone (1%) in Eucerin cream is applied 4–6 times a day.

   b. The importance of frequent application of a small amount, gently massaged into the affected area, must be emphasized.

3. Patient can use an antihistamine for antipruritic and sedative effect (see Tables 3-1 and 3-2 for dosage).

4. Secondary bacterial infection (beta-hemolytic streptococcal or staphylococcal) is common and must be treated before atopic dermatitis can be controlled. Consult physician.

VII. Complications

A. Secondary bacterial infection (beta-hemolytic streptococcal or staphylococcal).

B. Secondary viral infection (vaccinia or herpes simplex). Generalized vesiculopustular lesions develop; the patient can become seriously ill.

Table 3-2. Oral dosage of hydroxyzine HCl (Atarax, Vistaril) as an antipruritic and sedative.

Drug form	Body weight	Dose	Frequency
Hydroxyzine syrup[a] (Atarax) 10 mg per 5 ml[b]	8–10 kg (18–22 lbs)	2.5 ml	
	10–15 kg (22–23 lbs)	3.5 ml	
	15–20 kg (33–44 lbs)	5.0 ml	
	20–30 kg (44–66 lbs)	7.5 ml	
or			3 or 4 times a day
Hydroxyzine tablets[a] (Atarax) 10 mg per tablet	20–30 kg (44–66 lbs)	1 tablet	
	30–50 kg (66–110 lbs)	2 tablets	
or			
Hydroxyzine tablets[a] (Atarax) 25 mg per tablet	> 50 kg (110 lbs)	1 tablet	

[a]Caution: May cause drowsiness.
[b]Caution: Hydroxyzine *suspension* (Vistaril) is *25 mg per 5 ml.*

Note: Patients with atopic dermatitis and persons with whom they have close contact should *not* be vaccinated against smallpox.

VIII. Consultation-referral

   A. Secondary bacterial infection.

   B. Failure to respond to treatment within 2 weeks.

  IX. Follow-up. Return visit in 1 week, and periodically as needed.

Diaper Dermatitis

  I. Definition. Inflammation of the skin within the area usually covered by the diaper. It can be caused and aggravated by many factors acting separately or in combination, and a variety of morphologic changes can result.

 II. Etiology

   A. Contact irritants

     1. Urine irritation is probably caused by ammonia and other breakdown products.

      a. Diaper is not changed frequently enough.

      b. Occlusive plastic pants allow moisture and warmth to irritate and macerate skin.

     2. Stool

      a. Diaper is not changed frequently enough.

   b. Perineum is not cleaned thoroughly after defecation.

   c. Diarrhea.

   3. Chemicals. Detergents and soaps.

   4. Discharge (from vulvovaginitis).

B. Infection

   1. Bacterial. This is usually a secondary irritating colonization by a variety of organisms. Sometimes small staphylococcal furuncles are present.

   2. Fungal. *Candida albicans* organisms also may cause what is usually a secondary infection. It may be associated with oral candidiasis (thrush). Broad-spectrum antibiotic therapy (e.g., ampicillin) may cause candidiasis. Occasionally an infant acquires the infection from the hands of an adult contaminated with vaginal candidiasis.

   3. Viral. Vaccinia lesions may spread to the area of dermatitis.

C. Underlying skin disorder exaggerating the effects of contact irritation and infection.

   1. Seborrheic dermatitis.

   2. Atopic dermatitis.

III. Clinical features

A. Symptoms

   1. Sometimes, none.

   2. Pruritus.

   3. Irritability.

B. Signs

   1. Erythema is present, especially on the buttocks, genitalia, and lower abdomen.

   2. Erythematous papules, vesicles, and pustules as well as superficial ulcerations are present.

   3. Affected area may be moist and exudative.

   4. During healing of moderate to severe dermatitis, skin may be dry and scaly.

   5. *Candida* characteristically produces diffuse erythema that may be moist with satellite papules and pustules outside the margin of the erythema. The patient may also have oral candidiasis.

IV. Laboratory studies. Potassium hydroxide preparation of pustule contents or scraping of affected area, if candidiasis is suspected and morphology is not typical.

V. **Differential diagnosis.** None.

VI. **Treatment.** Advise parent to do the following:

A. **General treatment and prevention**

1. Keep diaper area dry and free from urine and stool:

   a. Change diapers frequently.

   b. Wash contaminated area with warm water at each diaper change. Use mild, nonperfumed, nonmedicated soap sparingly to avoid irritation.

   c. Allow air to circulate under diaper:

      (1) Use only one layer of diaper pinned loosely.

      (2) Do not put plastic pants over diaper.

      (3) Expose involved areas as much as possible to air.

2. Clean diapers well:

   a. Rinse thoroughly to remove soap.

   b. In the final rinse use a disinfectant (benzalkonium chloride [Zephiran] solution, 4 tablespoons per quart of water, or Diaparene).

B. **Mild inflammation (noncandidal)**

1. Follow general hygiene (see **A**).

2. Apply bland ointment after each diaper change (e.g., petrolatum, lanolin and petrolatum [A and D ointment], Diaparene).

C. **Moderate to severe inflammation (noncandidal)**

1. Follow general hygiene (see **A**).

2. For severe inflammation and weeping, apply aluminum acetate (Burow's) solution compresses for 20 minutes 3 times a day for 3–5 days only.

3. If there is no weeping, apply 1% hydrocortisone cream 4 times a day.

D. **Candidiasis**

1. Use good general hygiene (see **A**).

2. Apply nystatin (Mycostatin) cream liberally to affected area 3 times a day

   or

miconazole 2% (Micatin) or clotrimazole 1% (Lotrimin) to affected areas twice a day.

or

Apply Mycolog ointment (a combination of nystatin and triamicinolone) to affected area 2 or 3 times a day

or,

for stubborn cases, apply Lotrisone cream 2 or 3 times daily. (This medication should not be used for more than 2 weeks at any one time.)

3. If oral candidiasis is present or dermatitis is severe or recurrent, use nystatin (Mycostatin) oral suspension (100,000 units per milliliter) in a dosage of 2 ml orally 4 times a day for 1 week (1 ml in each side of mouth, not in the back of the throat, so that the medication is in contact with oral lesions as long as possible). It may be helpful to rub a portion of the dose on oral lesions with a cotton swab.

4. Examine mother for candidal vaginitis if infant has recurrent candidal diaper dermatitis.

VII. Complications

A. Spread to contiguous areas of abdomen and thighs.

B. Severe secondary bacterial infection.

VIII. Consultation-referral. Failure to respond to treatment within 1 week.

IX. Follow-up. Return visit in 1 week if there is no improvement.

Seborrheic Dermatitis: Pediatric and Adult

I. **Definition.** Oily, scaling condition affecting areas with large numbers of sebaceous glands (scalp, ears, central face, sternal area, and rarely, axillae and inguinal areas).

II. **Etiology.** Unknown.

III. **Clinical features**

A. **Symptoms**

1. Frequently, pruritis or flaking, or both.

2. Sometimes, no symptoms.

B. **Signs**

1. Usually, symmetric scaly eruption, often starting in scalp (cradle cap in infants).

   2. Progression to

   a. Eyebrows.

   b. Eyelids (scales around base of eyelashes).

   c. Nasolabial and postauricular folds, external auditory canal.

   d. Presternal area.

   e. Axillae and groin (rare).

   f. Diaper area in infants.

   3. Greasy scales, oily hair.

   4. Occasional association with acne.

   5. In infants, usually short-lived course without recurrence; in adults, tendency to recur.

IV. Laboratory studies. Potassium hydroxide preparation is negative in pure seborrhea; perform when diagnosis is in doubt or associated *Candida* infection is suspected.

V. Differential diagnosis

   A. Tinea capitis or corporis.

   B. Psoriasis.

   C. Contact dermatitis.

   D. Candidiasis.

VI. Treatment. Advise patient on the following measures:

   A. Adults

   1. Mild cases involving primarily the scalp

   a. Use any nonprescription dandruff shampoo containing selenium sulfide (e.g., Selsun Blue) or zinc pyrithione (e.g., Head & Shoulders, Sebulon) every 2–3 days (less often after symptoms subside). Lather, massage, and rinse well. Repeat sequence; leave second lather on scalp 6–10 minutes.

   b. If desired, use 2% sulfur and 2% salicylic acid cream twice a day on the skin.

   2. Severe cases

   a. Use one of these tar-containing shampoos every 2–3 days:

   (1) Sebutone.

   (2) Vanseb-T.

   (3) Ionil-T.

   (4) Pentrax.

    b. Apply 2% sulfur and 2% salicylic acid cream twice a day to affected areas.

    c. Apply a cortisone-containing lotion (1% hydrocortisone) to:

        (1) Scalp—twice a day for 10 days, then once a day for 7 days, then periodically as needed.

        (2) Other areas—once a day for 7–10 days, then as needed. Once the rash on the scalp is controlled, eruptions usually disappear from the face and ears.

B. Children

  1. Scalp

    a. Mild cases. Use any nonprescription shampoo. Lather, massage scalp with brush (soft brush for infant), and rinse well. Repeat sequence. Shampoo every other day until scales are gone, then twice a week.

    b. Extensive or thick scaling (cradle cap)

        (1) Use 2% sulfur and 2% salicylic acid shampoo (e.g., Sebulex). Lather, massage scalp with brush (soft brush for infant), and rinse well. Repeat sequence. Shampoo for next 2 days, then twice a week until scales are gone.

        (2) Use any nonprescription shampoo, with scalp massage, twice a week to prevent build-up of scales after using sulfur and salicylic acid shampoo treatment.

  2. Skin (oily skin with nonerythematous papules, as found on face and near hairline of infants)

    a. Wash twice a day with mild soap and water.

    b. Do not oil skin.

    c. Provide reassurance.

C. Erythema and scaling

  1. Examine potassium hydroxide preparation of scales if the affected area is moist and in diaper or intertriginous areas, to rule out candidiasis.

  2. Apply 1% hydrocortisone cream 4 times a day until dermatitis clears.

VII. Complications

  A. Secondary bacterial infection (usually beta-hemolytic streptococcal or staphylococcal).

  B. Candidal infection, especially in intertriginous, moist areas. Infection is more likely in obese patients.

C. Contact dermatitis from medicated shampoo or lotion.

VIII. Consultation-referral

A. Secondary bacterial infection.

B. No response to treatment.

IX. Follow-up. Return visit in 1 week if there is no improvement.

Folliculitis, Furuncles (Boils), Carbuncles: Pediatric and Adult

I. Definition

A. Folliculitis. A localized infection of a hair follicle. In areas of much hair (e.g., axilla), multiple infected follicles may be present.

B. Furuncle. A large, deep follicular infection with one drainage point.

C. Carbuncle. A large coalescence of furuncles with several drainage points, most commonly occurring in the back of the neck, the back, and thighs.

II. Etiology. *Staphylococcus aureus.* Preceding cutaneous trauma or lesion, immunologic deficiencies, diabetes, and nasal colonization with a virulent strain all predispose to infections.

III. Clinical features

A. Symptom. Pain. Tenderness, localized swelling.

B. Signs

1. Lesions vary in size from erythematous papules to large nodules with one or more drainage points.

2. Lesions are extremely tender, erythematous, and surrounded by inflammation.

3. Lesions initially are firm, but centers progress to become fluctuant.

4. Regional lymphadenitis may be present.

IV. Laboratory studies. There is no need to culture routinely in a patient without complicating disease or recurrences.

V. Differential diagnosis

A. Impetigo.

B. Foreign objects, with associated infection.

C. Insect bites.

VI. Treatment

A. **Folliculitis.** Tell the patient to wash affected area with soap and water and apply hot compresses for 20 minutes 4 times a day.

B. **Furuncles and carbuncles**

   1. Tell the patient to apply hot compresses for 20 minutes 4–6 times a day until fluctuant and ready for drainage.

   2. When fluctuant, have patient return for incision and drainage (after physician consultation).

   3. Pack cavity with iodoform or sterile gauze.

VII. **Complications**

   A. Usually, very few.

   B. Recurrences.

   C. Bacteremia, with metastatic infection.

VIII. **Consultation-referral**

   A. Carbuncles.

   B. Fever.

   C. Cellulitis or furuncles on the face.

IX. **Follow-up**

   A. **Folliculitis.** Return visit if lesions do not clear within a week.

   B. **Furuncle.** Return visit every other day until ready for drainage, then in 48 hours for dressing change. Further follow-up depends on size of lesion.

Herpes Simplex: Pediatric and Adult

I. **Definition.** A vesicular eruption of skin and mucous membranes appearing in two distinct clinical syndromes.

   A. **Herpes simplex labialis** ("of the lip") appears most often in children in its primary form and in adults in a less severe, recurrent form.

   B. **Herpes simplex progenitalis** appears as a primary and current problem in sexually active persons.

II. **Etiology.** Two similar but antigenically different strains of herpesvirus hominis:

   A. **Type 1** usually affects skin and mucous membranes above the umbilicus.

   B. **Type 2** usually affects skin and mucous membranes below the umbilicus. After the primary infection, the virus remains latent in cells that are in the area of the original lesions. (This is true of both types 1 and 2.)

Note: The difference in distribution between types 1 and 2 has become less distinct in recent years.

III. Clinical features

A. Type 1

1. **Primary infection (acute gingivostomatitis)** appears in persons not previously infected by the virus, usually children. The initial infection may be subclinical and asymptomatic or may appear as below.

   a. **Symptoms**

      (1) Soreness of the mouth and salivation.

      (2) Fever (as high as 105°F in children).

      (3) Malaise.

      (4) Course of 1–3 weeks.

   b. **Signs**

      (1) Vesicular eruption of gingival mucosa.

      (2) Breaking of vesicles, with grayish ulcerations.

      (3) Inflammation and swelling of gums and, sometimes, bleeding.

      (4) Usually, enlarged, tender submandibular lymph nodes.

      (5) Fever (as high as 105°F in children).

      (6) Infrequently, only tonsillar lesions.

2. **Recurrent infection**

   a. **Symptoms**

      (1) Burning and pain in affected area.

      (2) Generally, no systemic symptoms unless associated with another disease.

      (3) Reactivating factors, such as stress, physical trauma, sunlight, fever.

      (4) Course of about 10–14 days.

   b. **Signs.** Vesicles and ulcers, usually around vermilion border of lips.

B. Type 2

1. **Primary infection**

a. Symptoms

(1) Incubation period of 3–7 days.

(2) Mild to severe discomfort.

(3) Sometimes, prodrome of mild paresthesia or burning.

(4) Later, continuous vulval or penile pain, which may be severe.

(5) Dysuria and, occasionally, urinary retention.

(6) Tenderness of infected area.

(7) Sometimes, dyspareunia.

(8) Fever, headache, malaise.

(9) Course of 3–6 weeks.

b. Signs

(1) Indurated papules or vesicles surrounded by erythema, which often coalesce to form large ulcers.

(2) Location—vulva, genitocrural folds, perianal skin, vaginal and cervical mucosa in females, and urethral meatus and penis in males.

(3) Maceration in moist areas.

(4) With extensive involvement, edema is present.

(5) Inguinal lymphadenopathy.

(6) Low-grade fever.

(7) Sometimes, urethral discharge in males.

(8) A cluster of blisters or round erosions in the genital area.

2. Recurrent infection

a. Symptoms

(1) Symptoms are similar to those of the primary infection but usually less severe.

(2) Reactivation of the latent virus may be related to fever, emotional disturbance, premenstrual tension.

b. Signs

(1) Lesions are found in the same location as the primary infection.

(2) Signs tend to be less severe than those of the primary infection.

      (3) Early lesions are vesicles, which rupture and tend to ulcerate.

IV. Laboratory studies. Diagnosis is usually made on the basis of the clinical syndrome. Specific viral cultures, however, are now available to confirm the diagnosis.

V. Differential diagnosis

    A. Primary infection with herpesvirus type 1 may produce a generalized eruption that resembles chickenpox.

    B. Coxsackie and ECHO viruses cause herpangina, with papules, vesicles, and ulcers on the anterior tonsillar pillars, tonsils, soft palate, pharynx, and posterior buccal mucosa. If herpes simplex lesions begin posteriorly, as they occasionally do, they may be confused with herpangina.

    C. Lesions localized to the tonsils and pharynx may be confused with pharyngitis or tonsillitis of bacterial (most commonly streptococcal), viral, or mycoplasmal origin.

VI. Treatment. Advise patient on the following measures:

    A. Type 1

      1. Primary infection

        a. General measures

          (1) Take acetaminophen (Tylenol) or aspirin for pain or fever; see Chapter 5, Pharyngitis (Pediatric and Adult), **VI.C,** Table 5-5, p. 151, for dosage.

          (2) Use saline solution as mouthwash or for gargling.

          (3) Apply topical anesthetic, such as viscous lidocaine, to lesions as necessary.

          (4) Avoid contact with certain patients (see **VII.D**).

          (5) Maintain adequate fluid intake (especially children) to prevent dehydration. Use bland liquids (not citrus juices or carbonated drinks). Use straws to avoid lip, tongue, and gum lesions.

        b. Specific measures. None.

      2. Recurrence

        a. General measures

          (1) Apply a local drying or soothing agent (e.g., Blistex or Debrox) 3–4 times a day.

          (2) Avoid contact with certain patients (see **VII.D**).

b. Specific measures. NONE: A cyclovir is not approved for herpes labialis.

B. Type 2

1. Primary infection

a. General measures

(1) Take acetaminophen (Tylenol) or aspirin (see pp. 150–151).

(2) Take sitz baths in tepid water as often as necessary.

(3) Use a topical anesthetic, such as dibucaine HCl (Nupercaine), if pain is intense. Generally, however, topical anesthetics are to be avoided because of the potential for allergic reactions.

(4) Avoid contact with certain patients (see **VII.D**).

(5) Avoid sexual intercourse until lesions heal.

b. Specific measures. Apply acyclovir 5% ointment (Zovirax) to lesions every 3 hours (six times daily) for one week. Use a finger cot or rubber glove when applying to prevent autoinoculation and transmission to other persons.

or

In severe cases, give acyclovir (Zovirax) 200 mg tablets orally every 4 hours, while awake (five times daily) for 10 days. (Consult Physician).

2. Recurrent infection. Intermittent or chronic suppressive therapy with oral acyclovir (Zovirax) may be indicated in recurrent episodes. Consult physician.

VII. Complications

A. Involvement of other parts of the body:

1. Conjunctivitis.

2. Keratitis.

3. Generalized vesicular eruption.

B. Secondary bacterial infection (beta-hemolytic streptococcal or staphylococcal, or both) of skin lesions.

C. Dehydration in infants and younger children with gingivostomatitis and poor fluid intake.

D. Spread to patients at risk of developing disseminated and severe herpes simplex. Isolate from the following:

1. Patients with open skin lesions, such as burns and dermatitis.

2. Newborns.

3. Patients on immunosuppressive therapy.

VIII. Consultation-referral

A. Conjunctivitis.

B. Keratitis.

C. Persistent headache and vomiting, photophobia, convulsions, or neurologic findings suggestive of encephalitis.

D. Infection in late pregnancy because of risk to newborn, in whom fatal disseminated disease can develop.

E. Severe primary infection (type 1 or 2).

F. Very poor oral fluid intake (usually in infants and younger children).

G. Secondary bacterial infection.

IX. Follow-up. Return visit in 1 week if no improvement or if any of the following develops:

A. Eye symptoms.

B. Secondary bacterial infection.

C. Inadequate fluid intake.

Herpes Zoster (Shingles): Pediatric and Adult

I. Definition. Usually, a unilateral vesicular eruption distributed along the dermatomes of infected nerve roots. It is thought to be due to reactivation of a latent viral infection.

II. Etiology

A. Herpes zoster is caused by a virus that appears to be the same as the chickenpox virus.

B. Certain patients, particularly those with altered immune responses, have an increased tendency toward development of herpes zoster. They include:

1. Patients with lymphomas, especially Hodgkin's disease.

2. Patients on corticosteroids.

3. Patients on other immunosuppressive agents.

4. Patients with disseminated malignancies.

III. Clinical features

A. Symptoms

1. Fever.

2. Pain, occasionally quite severe, along a dermatome. (Pain may begin as long as 3–5 days before the rash begins.) Children may not have pain.

B. Signs

1. Eruption begins with red macules; progresses sequentially to papules, vesicles, pustules, and crusts; and resolves over 1–2 weeks.

2. Vesicles appear in clumps over the first week.

3. Involvement is unilateral.

4. Pain and eruption follow a dermatomic pattern.

5. The thoracic and cervical nerve roots are most often affected.

IV. Laboratory studies. Tzanck prep is available in some labs.

V. Differential diagnosis

A. **Pain appearing before rash.** Diagnosis is difficult in this situation, and the differential diagnosis must include any cause of pain localized to the area in question. (After rash develops, the distribution and appearance of herpes zoster are typical.)

B. **Impetigo**

C. **Herpes simplex**

VI. Treatment. Advise patient on the following measures:

A. General therapy

1. Take acetaminophen (Tylenol) or aspirin for fever or pain; see Chapter 5, Pharyngitis (Pediatric and Adult), **VI.C,** Table 5-5, p. 151, for dosage.

2. If needed, use a narcotic for pain. Consult physician.

3. Use cool water or aluminum acetate (Burow's) solution soaks for vesicles or crusts.

4. Avoid contact with patients listed in **II.B.**

B. **Specific therapy.** Oral and intravenous Zovirax therapy is now available (consult physician).

VII. Complications

A. Dissemination

1. Occurs in more than 50% of patients with Hodgkin's disease.

2. Rarely occurs in patients without underlying immunologic problems.

B. Bacterial superinfection

C. Postherpetic neuralgia (continued pain in dermatome site after rash has disappeared). Occurs more frequently in persons over 50.

VIII. Consultation-referral

A. Any patient on steroids or other immunosuppressive drugs or over 50.

B. Coexisting Hodgkin's disease or other malignancy.

C. Symptoms persisting beyond 2 weeks.

D. Bacterial superinfection.

E. Ocular involvement.

IX. Follow-up. Return visit if there is no improvement within 2 weeks.

Impetigo: Pediatric and Adult

I. Definition. A condition involving the superficial layers of the skin characterized by seropurulent vesicles surrounded by an erythematous base.

II. Etiology and epidemiology

A. Impetigo is caused by either group: beta-hemolytic streptococci, or Coagulase-positive staphylococci. Occasionally, both organisms may be found.

B. It may be spread by direct contact with infected persons and possibly by insects, or it may be secondary to infections of the upper respiratory tract.

C. Incubation period is 2–10 days.

D. The untreated patient is contagious until the lesions are healed; treatment shortens the period of contagiousness.

E. Impetigo may be a complication of insect bites, abrasions, or dermatitis.

F. Peak incidence is in late summer and early fall.

G. Impetigo is most common in infants and children.

III. Clinical features

A. Symptoms

1. Constitutional symptoms are unusual unless lesions are widespread.

2. Itching is common.

B. Signs

1. Superficial vesicles are present, containing serous fluid that be comes purulent and surrounded by areas of erythema.

2. Pustules rupture, dry centrally, and form a honey-colored crust.

3. Lesions vary in size from a few millimeters to several centi meters.

IV. **Laboratory studies.** If the diagnosis is in doubt, culture fluid from an intact vesicle or pustule or the base of a lesion after the crust is removed.

V. **Differential diagnosis**

A. Noninfected insect bites.

B. Herpes simplex.

C. Chickenpox.

D. Other vesicular or ulcerating skin lesions.

VI. **Treatment**

A. Advise patient to do the following:

1. Soak and then gently scrub lesions with warm water and soap three times a day to soften and remove crusts. Be careful not to spread infection to family members by contaminated clothes and towels.

2. Trim fingernails to prevent further spread.

B. Use antibiotic therapy for all patients with more than a few le sions; there is some debate among authorities about the use of penicillin for treatment of patients with one or two small lesions (Antibiotic therapy will promote healing, decreasing the period of contagiousness and therefore the spread of impetigo.) It is not known whether early treatment of streptococcal impetigo will de crease the incidence of secondary nephritis.

1. Benzathine penicillin G (Bicillin, long-acting). (Ask whether pa tient is allergic to penicillin.)

a. Patients weighing less than 25 kg (55 lb)—one IM injection of 600,000 units.

b. Patients weighing more than 25 kg (55 lb)—one IM injection of 1,200,000 units.

Note: Patients should be observed by health care provider for at least 20 minutes after receiving an injection.

or

2. Oral penicillin (children and adults)—penicillin V, 250 mg 3 times a day for 10 days. (Ask whether patient is allergic to pen icillin.)

Table 3-3. Oral dosage of erythromycin ethylsuccinate suspension (200 mg per 5 ml)

Body weight	Dose	Frequency
6–9 kg (13–20 lb)	160 mg (4 ml)	
9–12 kg (20–26 lb)	240 mg (6 ml)	
12–16 kg (26–35 lb)	320 mg (8 ml)	
16–20 kg (35–44 lb)	400 mg (10 ml)	2 times a day for 10 days
20–24 kg (44–53 lb)	480 mg (12 ml)	
24–28 kg (53–62 lb)[a]	560 mg (14 ml)	
28–32 kg (62–70 lb)[a]	640 mg (16 ml)	
Over 32 kg (over 70 lb)[a]	800 mg (20 ml)	

[a]Patients weighing over 25 kg (over 55 lb) may be given erythromycin base tablets (250 mg per tablet), 500 mg (2 tablets) twice a day for 10 days taken 1 hour before meals.
Note: If abdominal discomfort develops, divide dose in half and give 4 times a day.

or

   3. If patient is allergic to penicillin, use erythromycin as directed in Table 3-3.

 C. In cases where lesions are predominantly bullous, the organism is more likely to be staphylococcus aureus, and should be treated with: erythromycin (40–50 mg/kg/d divided into 4 doses) or dicloxacillin (12–25 mg/kg/d divided into 4 doses).

 D. Treat all people in close contact with patient, who have impetiginous lesions, as soon as possible to avoid reinfection and further spread.

VII. Complications

 A. Acute glomerulonephritis may follow infection if the strain of streptococcus is nephritogenic.

 B. Acute rheumatic fever is *not* a complication.

VIII. Consultation-referral

 A. Failure to resolve.

 B. Presence of acute glomerulonephritis in the community.

IX. Follow-up

 A. Clinic visit if no improvement within 1 week.

 B. Clinic visit for persons in close contact with the patient, who have impetiginous lesions, as soon as possible.

Candidiasis: Adult

I. **Definition.** An infection of the skin caused by the fungus *Candida albicans.*

II. **Etiology.** *C. albicans.*

III. **Clinical features**

   A. **Symptoms**

   1. Itching.

   2. Burning pain, particularly with vulval involvement.

   3. Frequent association with diabetes mellitus, particularly when diabetes is uncontrolled. Therefore, inquire about polyuria, polydipsia, and polyphagia.

   4. Occasional association with use of birth control pills.

   B. **Signs**

   1. An erythematous macular rash is seen, usually involving intertriginous areas and vulva and sometimes becoming confluent with satellite lesions (inguinal creases and scrotum in males).

   2. Vulval rash, with white, cheesy exudate, is usually associated with candidal vaginitis. Exudate may also appear in intertriginous areas.

IV. **Laboratory studies**

   A. Potassium hydroxide preparation of the lesion is positive for *Candida.*

   B. Culture of organisms should be obtained when the diagnosis is in doubt.

   C. The level of urine or blood sugar, or both, should be measured to evaluate possible diabetes mellitus.

V. **Differential diagnosis**

   A. Seborrheic dermatitis.

   B. Other fungal skin infections.

VI. **Treatment**

   A. **Coexisting diabetes.** In a diabetic patient, candidiasis *cannot* be controlled or cured until the diabetes is controlled. Therefore, diabetes must be evaluated and properly managed by a physician.

   B. **Intertriginous candidiasis.** Use one of the following two times daily:

1. Miconazole (Micatin) 2% cream,

   or

2. Clotrimazole (Lotrimin, Mycelex) 1% cream,

   or

3. Nystatin (Mycostatin) cream.

C. **Candidal vulvovaginitis.** Advise patient on the following measures:

1. Apply aluminum acetate (Burow's) solution compresses or Mycolog ointment, or both, to vulval lesions twice a day if they are moist or markedly inflamed.

2. Vaginal treatment with: a. Miconazole nitrate 2% (Monistat) vaginal cream, 1 applicator nightly for 3 days, or b. Clotrimazole 1% (Gyne-Lotrimin) vaginal cream or suppositories, 1 dose nightly for 7 days, or c. Miconazole 100 mg. vaginal tablets (Monistat-3), 1 tablet nightly for 3 days.

3. Avoid contamination from gastrointestinal tract (instruct patient in proper toiletry).

4. Use Mycostatin oral tablets in resistant cases.

5. In recurrent cases, the male sexual partner may need to be treated for intertriginous candidiasis.

6. For resistant cases, oral Ketoconazole (Nizoral) is now available (consult physician).

VII. **Complications.** None.

VIII. **Consultation-referral.** Failure to resolve in 2 weeks.

IX. **Follow-up.** Once a week until resolution occurs.

Pityriasis Rosea: Pediatric and Adult

I. **Definition.** A self-limiting, mild, scaly skin eruption occurring primarily in adolescents and young adults and lasting from 3–6 weeks.

II. **Etiology.** Unknown. (Possibly a hypersensitivity reaction to a viral infection.)

III. **Clinical features**

A. **Symptoms**

1. Pruritus—usually mild, sometimes intense.

2. Occasionally, mild malaise.

    3. Occasionally, symptoms of a mild upper respiratory tract infection.

B. Signs

    1. The herald patch is the initial lesion in most cases, but it may not be present or may go unnoticed. It presents as a 4- to 5-cm round or oval scaling erythematous plaque occurring anywhere on body.

    2. The herald patch is followed in several days to a week by multiple small 1- to 2-cm maculopapular lesions that are pale red and round or oval, with a wrinkled surface and peripheral rim of small, fine scales. These lesions occur in crops over the trunk and proximal extremities and tend to occur with their long axis oriented in the direction of the skin cleavage planes parallel to the ribs.

IV. Laboratory studies. Serologic test for syphilis to rule out secondary syphilis.

V. Differential diagnosis

    A. Secondary syphilis.

    B. Seborrhea.

    C. Tinea versicolor.

VI. Treatment. Usually, none. Drying lotions (e.g., calamine lotion) may relieve the itching. Oral antihistamines, either diphenhydramine (Benadryl) or hydroxyzine (Atarax, Vistaril), may also be helpful; see Tables 3-1 and 3-2, pp. 96–97, for dosage. Inform the patient that the rash will last several weeks but is self-limited.

VII. Complications. None.

VIII. Consultation-referral. None.

IX. Follow-up. Return visit as needed.

Contact Dermatitis Due to Poison Oak or Poison Ivy: Pediatric and Adult

    I. Definition. An acute dermatitis resulting from contact with the resin of poison oak or poison ivy.

    II. Etiology. Most cases from contact with the leaves of the plant; however, cases may come from digging in ground that contains the growing plant. An outbreak may also result from contact with the smoke of burning plants, unwashed contaminated clothes, dried (uprooted plants that still retain resin, or a pet that has had contact with the plant.

III. Clinical features

A. Pruritic vesicles usually appear on the extremities.

B. Early eruption may be erythematous and raised without vesicles.

C. Linear streaks of erythema or vesicles are usually seen where plant has brushed across skin.

IV. Laboratory studies. None.

V. Differential diagnosis

A. Other contact dermatitides.

B. Insect bites.

VI. Treatment

A. Advise patient on the following preventive measures:

  1. Be familiar with the appearance of the plant and how to avoid it.

  2. Wash all clothes worn at the time of contact.

  3. If known exposure occurs in the future, immediately wash contact area to prevent or minimize clinical symptoms.

B. General measures. Tell patient to do the following:

  1. Soak the affected area in saline or aluminum acetate (Burow's) solution if this can be done easily, or use cold compresses for 20 minutes 4–6 times a day. This is the mainstay of therapy.

  2. Apply a drying lotion (e.g., calamine lotion) after each soak or cold compress.

  3. Avoid topical lotions containing antihistamine or benzocaine derivatives. These ingredients add nothing, and may act as allergens.

  4. Use an oral antihistamine for sedation and as an antipruritic in moderate to severe cases (see Tables 3-1 and 3-2, pp. 96–97, for dosage).

  5. If there is no weeping, apply 1% hydrocortisone cream 4–6 times a day.

  6. Use an oral steroid after consultation for severe cases and cases involving the eyes, face, mucous membranes, and genitalia.

VII. Complications. Secondary bacterial infections; see Impetigo (Pediatric and Adult, pp. 111–113).

VIII. Consultation-referral

  A. Widespread involvement or marked discomfort, or both.

  B. Involvement of the eyes or other sensitive areas, such as oral mucous membranes and genitalia.

IX. Follow-up. Return visit in 3 days if there is no improvement.

Scabies: Pediatric and Adult

I. Definition. An intensely pruritic rash caused by the mite *Sarcoptes scabiei.*

II. Etiology

  A. The initial lesion is a burrow ½–2 cm in length, with a papule or vesicle at its blind end, not associated with itching. After several days, sensitivity to the mite results in severe pruritus followed by punctate excoriations from scratching and impetiginous and eczematous changes at the site of the lesion. A generalized urticarial rash may also develop.

  B. The mite is transferred by personal contact, does not live long in clothing or bedding, and is found in association with poor personal hygiene and crowded living conditions.

III. Clinical features

  A. Symptom. Pruritus (most severe at night).

  B. Signs

   1. The characteristic burrow appears as a thin line ½–2 cm in length, ending in a papule or vesicle. Unfortunately, this sign is not seen in many patients.

   2. Characteristic locations of lesions:

   a. Men

   (1) Interdigital folds, wrists (85% of cases).

   (2) Elbows, genitalia, ankles, feet (40% of cases).

   b. Women

   (1) Palms and nipples (most frequent sites).

   (2) Other sites (see **a**).

   c. Children

   (1) Palms.

   (2) Soles of feet.

      (3) Head.

      (4) Neck.

      (5) Legs.

      (6) Buttocks.

   3. Secondary changes:

     a. Excoriation.

     b. Pustules and crusts of secondary bacterial infection.

     c. Eczema with weeping or scaling, or both.

IV. Laboratory studies. Attempt to isolate the mite by scraping a burrow, papule, or vesicle and placing the specimen in mineral oil (on a slide) and examine microscopically. (Potassium hydroxide preparation is not used, because it destroys the characteristic feces.)

V. Differential diagnosis. Scabies may take many forms and be confused with:

  A. Impetigo.

  B. Eczema.

  C. Urticaria.

VI. Treatment. Advise patient on these treatment measures:

  A. Specific agents

    1. For children under 3 years of age use 10% precipitated sulfur in petrolatum nightly for 3 nights. Apply to child's entire body from the neck down, with special attention to hands, feet, and intertriginous areas. Treatment is preceded by warm soap and water bath using a soft brush. A bath may be taken before reapplying medication and 24 hours after the third application.

    2. For adults and children over 3 years of age use:

      a. Gamma benzene hexachloride 1% (Kwell), cream or lotion, applied to entire body from the neck down, not just to obvious lesions, with special attention to hands, feet, and intertriginous areas. Keep away from eyes and mucous membranes. Treatment is preceded by a warm soap and water bath using a soft brush and is followed by drying with a towel. Medication is thoroughly removed in 8 hours by a bath similar to the first.

    Note: Effects of Kwell on the central nervous system, including convulsions, have been associated with applying the drug too frequently or leaving it on the skin longer than recommended. Therefore, no more than necessary should be prescribed (30 gm or 1 ounce for an average adult), and patients should be cautioned against overuse.

or

b. Crotamiton 10% (Eurax) cream, applied to entire body from neck down, as above for Kwell. A second coat should be applied in 24 hours and the patient should bathe 48 hours past the last application. With correct use, crotamiton has very few side effects; slight local irritation occurs occasionally. Crotamiton has antipruritic properties as well as scabicidal effects.

or

c. Precipitated sulfur (10%) in petrolatum (see **VI.A.1**).

B. Hygiene. Underclothing, pajamas, sheets, and pillowcases should be washed with boiling water, laundered, and ironed, or washed by machine using hot cycle.

C. Members of the household and sexual contacts with scabies should be treated at the same time.

D. An oral antihistamine, such as diphenhydramine HCl (Benadryl) or hydroxyzine HCl (Atarax, Vistaril) may be helpful to relieve itching (see Tables 3-1 and 3-2 for dosage, pp. 96–97).

VII. Complications

A. Secondary bacterial infection.

B. Eczema.

C. Reaction to gamma benzene hexachloride (Kwell):

1. Dermatitis.

2. CNS toxicity.

D. Inappropriate treatment with topical corticosteroids may worsen the infestation.

VIII. Consultation-referral

A. Failure to respond to therapy.

Note: Following effective therapy, signs and symptoms may persist for several weeks due to hypersensitivity reaction to the mite, not necessarily to treatment failure.

B. Absence of characteristic burrows or papules.

C. Eczema.

D. Secondary bacterial infection.

IX. Follow-up. Patient should return if not cured by therapy, or if disease recurs.

Tinea Corporis (Ringworm of Nonhairy Skin): Pediatric and Adult

I. **Definition.** Superficial fungal infection involving the trunk or limbs. (For fungal infection of the feet, see Tinea Pedis [Athlete's Foot] [Pediatric and Adult]. Refer all fungal infections of the scalp to a physician.)

II. **Etiology.** Several different fungi.

III. **Clinical features**

   A. **Symptoms.** Condition is asymptomatic or mildly pruritic.

   B. **Signs**

   1. Erythematous, scaling patches (usually one or two) that are round or oval are seen. The lesions start small, then expand outward, with clearing of the eruption in the center of the patch and activity restricted to the border of the lesion (hence the name *ringworm*). The border of the lesion is usually raised and scaly.

   2. Lesions are most common on the face and arms.

IV. **Laboratory studies**

   A. Potassium hydroxide (KOH) preparation of scales from the active border is positive for hyphae. (Scales from the center of a lesion may be negative.)

   B. Fungal culture is a more sensitive test but takes 1–2 weeks for results. It need not be done with a typical lesion.

V. **Differential diagnosis**

   A. **Candidal infection.** This is usually intertriginous and redder than ringworm. It has less tendency toward central clearing, and satellite lesions are present outside the main lesion.

   B. **Pityriasis rosea.** The herald patch may mimic ringworm, but it is KOH-negative. Pityriasis lesions also have a more widespread distribution. Look for other pityriasis lesions elsewhere.

   C. **Seborrheic dermatitis.** Lesions are usually not round or oval, and they are KOH-negative. When lesions are on the face, differentiation is very difficult. In contrast to seborrheic dermatitis, fungal infections will not clear with topical steroid treatment.

VI. **Treatment.** If thickening of skin has occurred, treatment with a topical antifungal agent may require 2–3 weeks or longer. Instruct patient to apply one of the following twice daily after soap and water washing and thorough drying of the lesion: Continue application for at least 2 weeks.

    A. Tolnaftate 1% (Tinactin), cream or solution,

      or

    B. Miconazole nitrate 2% (MicaTin), cream or lotion.

      or

    C. Clotrimazole 1% (Lotrimin), cream or solution.

VII. Complications

    A. Secondary bacterial infection.

    B. Allergy to topical antifungal agent.

VIII. Consultation-referral

    A. Severe or widespread infection.

    B. Infection of the scalp.

    C. Secondary bacterial infection.

    D. Failure to respond to treatment.

  IX. Follow-up. Return visit in 2 weeks if there is no significant improvement.

Tinea Pedis (Athlete's Foot): Pediatric and Adult

  I. Definition. A pruritic cracking and peeling eruption of the feet, especially the toe webs.

 II. Etiology. Several different fungi.

III. Clinical features

    A. Symptom. Intense itching is characteristic but not always present.

    B. Signs

      1. Eruptions usually start between the toes and occasionally spread to the soles or sides or even the tops of the feet.

      2. Vesicles are occasionally present.

      3. Toenails may be thickened, with debris under the nail.

      4. Hands and groin may show evidence of fungal infection.

IV. Laboratory studies

    A. Potassium hydroxide (KOH) preparation of scales or the top of vesicles for typical hyphae is optional.

    B. Fungal culture may be positive when the KOH preparation is negative, but need not be done with typical lesions.

V. Differential diagnosis

    A. Contact dermatitis (shoe leather dye, nylon, soap, etc.).

    B. Secondary syphilis.

    C. Psoriasis.

    D. Dyshidrosis.

    E. Neurodermatitis.

    F. Candidiasis.

    G. Bacterial infection.

    H. Reiter's disease.

VI. Treatment. Advise patient on the following measures:

    A. General measures

        1. Thoroughly dry interdigital areas after bathing.

        2. Use absorbent cotton socks.

        3. Change socks at least once a day.

    B. Specific measures

        1. Soak the feet in aluminum acetate (Burow's) solution or tap water 20–30 minutes twice a day if vesicles are present.

          Then

        2. Apply an antifungal agent; see Tinea Corporis (Ringworm of Nonhairy Skin) (Pediatric and Adult), **VI,** pp. 121–122.

VII. Complications

    A. Secondary bacterial infection.

    B. Allergy to topical antifungal agent.

VIII. Consultation-referral

    A. Secondary bacterial infection.

    B. No response to topical antifungal agents or worsening of condition after treatment has started.

    C. Fungal infection elsewhere on the body.

IX. Follow-up. Return visit in 3–5 days if there is no improvement.

Tinea Versicolor: Pediatric and Adult

    I. Definition. Benign, chronic, asymptomatic, superficial fungal infection.

    II. Etiology. The fungus *Malassezia furfur.*

III. Clinical features

A. Symptom. The patient shows concern about his or her appearance.

B. Signs

1. White, pink, tan, or brown macular spots, patches, or large con-fluent lesions are present, located mainly on the upper trunk, front and back. The lesions may extend to the abdomen and upper extremities, and less commonly to the neck and face.

2. Light scratching produces fine scales.

3. Infected areas do not tan when exposed to sunlight and appear much lighter than surrounding skin. In winter they may appear darker than surrounding areas.

IV. Laboratory studies. Potassium hydroxide (KOH) preparation of scales reveals clusters of round spoors, and filaments.

V. Differential diagnosis

A. Seborrheic dermatitis.

B. Vitiligo.

C. Pityriasis alba, if lesions are on the face.

VI. Treatment

A. Counseling. The patient should be told that:

1. Recurrence is very common.

2. The condition is benign even without treatment.

3. Although the infection is eradicated with treatment and scaling stops, the hypopigmented areas will remain until tanned by ex-posure to the sun or until the surrounding tanned area fades.

B. Specific measures. Advise patient on these measures:

1. Bathe or shower in the evening, scrubbing lesions with a stiff brush.

2. Apply selenium sulfide 2.5% (Selsun, Exsel) to entire body (re-gardless of location of rash) from neck down to knees and wrists, avoiding genital area. Allow it to remain for several hours or overnight. Repeat application in 1 week.

VII. Complications. Irritation from selenium sulfide if it is in contact with the eyes or anogenital area.

VII. Consultation-referral. No improvement after treatment and after skin color has had an opportunity to return to normal.

IX. Follow-up. Return visit as desired by patient.

Urticaria (Hives): Pediatric and Adult

I. **Definition.** Pruritic, red, raised plaques or welts, usually representing an allergic reaction.

II. **Etiology.** Urticaria is an allergic reaction, usually to drugs (oral and injected), foods, insect bites, inhalants, or injections. Occasionally it is due to an infection (e.g., herpes simplex, upper respiratory tract infection, tooth abscess, urinary tract infection). No cause is found in many cases.

III. **Clinical features**

A. **Symptoms**

1. Itching.

2. Occasionally, stinging or paresthesia.

B. **Signs**

1. Red, raised plaques or welts with sharp borders are present, usually on the trunk and extremities. They vary in number and size.

2. Lesions usually fade in less than 12 hours, sometimes in 20–30 minutes. If lesions persist (in the same location) for more than 24 hours, the diagnosis is often erythema multiforme or multiple insect bites.

•3. The chest is clear to auscultation, and the patient is not wheezing.

IV. **Laboratory studies.** None.

V. **Differential diagnosis**

A. Erythema multiforme.

B. Cutaneous manifestation of anaphylaxis.

C. Multiple insect bites.

D. Contact dermatitis.

E. Acute exanthem.

VI. **Treatment**

A. If clinical features of anaphylaxis are present, institute immediate specific treatment; see Chapter 2, Anaphylaxis (Pediatric and Adult), **VI,** pp. 56–57.

B. For widespread urticaria and intense pruritis or angioedema, inject aqueous epinephrine, 1:1000, subcutaneously.

Table 3-4. Oral dosage of chlorpheniramine maleate (Chlor-Trimeton)

Body weight	Dose	Frequency
10–20 kg (22–44 lb)	2.5 ml	
20–30 kg (44–66 lb)	5 ml (½ tablet)	4 times a day
30–40 kg (66–88 lb)	5–7.5 ml (½ tablet)	
Over 40 kg (over 88 lb)	5–10 ml (½–1 tablet)	

1. **Pediatric dose.** 0.01 ml per kg (0.005 ml per lb); maximum dose, 0.3 ml.

2. **Adult dose.** 0.3–0.5 ml.

Note: It may be necessary to repeat the dose every 1–2 hours for several doses.

C. Use an oral antihistamine for less severe urticaria and after injection of epinephrine (**B**).

1. Diphenhydramine HCl (see Table 3-1, p. 96, for dosage).

    or

2. Chlorpheniramine maleate (Chlor-Trimeton) syrup, 2 mg per 5 ml; or tablets, 4 mg per tablet (see Table 3-4 for dosage).

    or

3. Hydroxyzine HCl (Atarax, Vistaril) (see Table 3-2, p. 97, for dosage).

D. Search carefully for offending agent and eliminate or avoid it. Inquire about diet history, drug history, insect bites.

E. Provide additional antipruritic effect, if necessary:

1. Soak in a tub of cool water.

2. Add colloidal oatmeal (Aveeno) to bath water.

VII. Complications

A. Systemic reaction to allergen (e.g., anaphylaxis or serum sickness).

B. Drowsiness secondary to antihistamine therapy. Patients must be cautioned about activities requiring alertness (e.g., driving motor vehicles).

VIII. Consultation-referral

A. Evidence of edema of the larynx (hoarseness, inspiratory stridor).

B. Evidence of anaphylaxis (hypotension, tachycardia, paroxysmal coughing, severe anxiety, dyspnea, wheezing, vomiting, cyanosis). Treat immediately as anaphylaxis; see Chapter 2, Anaphylaxis (Pediatric and Adult), **VI,** pp. 56–57.

C. Chronic or recurrent urticaria lasting more than 1 week.

IX. Follow-up

A. The patient should return in 48 hours if lesions persist or new signs or symptoms develop.

B. If urticaria was caused by an insect sting, patient should be referred for hyposensitization.

Warts: Pediatric and Adult

I. Definition. An intradermal papilloma most frequently appearing in three distinct clinical patterns:

A. Common warts.

B. Plantar warts.

C. Venereal warts.

II. Etiology. Human papilloma virus.

III. Clinical features

A. Common warts

1. **Symptoms.** Generally, none.

2. **Signs.** Small, circular skin-colored to gray-brown papillomas. These generally appear on the hand and fingers, but may appear anywhere on the skin or mucous membranes.

B. Plantar warts

1. **Symptoms.** Plantar warts may cause severe pain with walking or standing.

2. **Signs.** These warts resemble corns or calluses, with a central nodule containing several punctate spots.

C. Venereal warts

1. **Symptoms.** Usually, none.

2. **Signs.** Small papillomas are seen on the foreskin and penis in males (particularly those who are uncircumcised) and on the perineum and vaginal mucosa in females.

IV. Laboratory studies. None.

V. Differential diagnosis

A. Corns, calluses.

B. Melanoma.

VI. Treatment

A. Common warts. Apply dichloroacetic acid every 1–2 weeks. A crust will form; this should be removed at each visit and the lesion retreated. Alternative treatments involving freezing with liquid nitrogen and other modalities are available (consult physician).

B. Plantar warts

   1. Pare down callus with scalpel and apply dichloroacetic acid as directed in **A.**

   or

   2. Apply a salicylic paint (e.g., Wart-Off, Duofilm) to wart (avoid surrounding skin) once or twice daily. Treatment may be continued for up to four weeks.

   or

   Apply a 40% salicylic acid plaster.

     a. Cover the callus with plaster and bandage with tape.

     b. Remove in 5–7 days and pare down callus and wart.

     c. Treatment may be repeated, but if tenderness intervenes, wait until it subsides.

C. Venereal warts. Apply 20–25% podophyllum resin in tincture of benzoin.

   1. Coat area around wart with petrolatum to prevent spread of podophyllum to uninvolved area.

   2. Coat warts with podophyllum mixture.

   3. Allow podophyllum to remain 3–5 hours. (Use a shorter time initially, increasing the length of time with later application.)

   4. Instruct patient to take a sitz bath after 3–5 hours.

   5. Inform the patient that the lesions may be painful for several days.

   6. Repeat the treatment at weekly intervals until warts are gone.

   7. Treat any coexisting vaginitis (see guidelines in Chapter 14, pp. 316–320).

VII. Complications

A. Tenderness may occur around treated area.

B. Overtreatment may lead to scarring.

VIII. Consultation-referral

A. Large numbers of warts or large warts (which are best treated by other methods).

B. Resistance to therapy.

C. Venereal warts involving anus.

IX. Follow-up. As often as necessary for treatment.

Disorders of the Eye

4

Conjunctivitis: Pediatric and Adult

I. **Definition.** Inflammation of the eyelid or bulbar conjunctiva, or both.

II. **Etiology**

A. **Bacterial infection**

1. Pneumococcus, staphylococcus aureus, streptococcus, hemophilus influenzae, and others.

2. Gonococcus, especially in the first month of life. If the infection is contracted during birth, onset will be at age 3–5 days.

B. **Viral infection**

1. Adenoviruses: adenopharyngeal conjunctivitis (APC) and epidemic keratoconjunctivitis (EKC) are most frequently found. EKC is highly contagious and proper hand washing is especially important to prevent hand-to-eye spread. Towels and tonometers have been implicated.

2. Associated with an upper respiratory tract infection.

3. Conjunctivitis with epidemic sore throat, high fever, and preauricular and submandibular adenitis, usually due to an adenovirus.

4. Inclusion blennorrhea, occurring in newborns and during childhood from contaminated swimming pools.

5. Vaccinia, herpesvirus hominis type 1 (herpes simplex), herpes zoster. Lesions are usually present on the skin also.

C. **Allergic reaction.** Conjunctivitis is often associated with seasonal allergic rhinitis, which is usually due to pollen allergy.

D. **Foreign body or trauma**

E. **Chemical irritants**

F. **Systemic infection**

    1. Measles.

    2. Rocky Mountain spotted fever.

III. Clinical features

A. Symptoms

    1. Mild irritation.

    2. Mild photophobia.

    3. Excessive lacrimation.

    4. Normal vision.

B. Signs

    1. Infected conjunctiva.

    2. Discharge

        a. Purulent in bacterial infection.

        b. Mucopurulent in viral infection (occasionally becoming secondarily infected with bacteria).

        c. Mucoid and stringy or watery in allergic reaction.

        d. Watery when caused by a foreign body, air pollution, allergy.

    3. Sometimes, conjunctival edema.

    4. Clear cornea.

    5. Pupils are normal in size and react to light.

    6. Enlarged preauricular nodes.

IV. Laboratory studies. Culture of exudate for gonococcus in first month of life.

V. Differential diagnosis

A. Lacrimal duct obstruction. This is a congenital disorder seen in the first few months of life as overflow tearing and secondary bacterial infection of obstructed duct, with persistent purulent discharge.

B. Acute iritis (see Table 4-1, p. 132) and iridocyclitis

C. Acute glaucoma. See Table 4-1.

D. Blepharitis

VI. Treatment

A. Consultation on specific cases (see VIII).

B. Allergic conjunctivitis, if acute and mild, will respond to treatment of accompanying allergic rhinitis; see Chapter 5, Allergic Rhinitis (Pediatric and Adult), pp. 145–149.

Table 4-1. Differential diagnosis of three eye disorders

Parameter	Acute conjunctivitis	Acute iritis	Acute glaucoma
Pain	Mild discomfort	Moderate pain, with photophobia	Moderate to severe pain, with nausea and vomiting
Vision	Normal	Slightly to moderately blurred	Very blurred
Discharge	Often mucopurulent	Clear	Clear
Cornea	Clear	Clear	Cloudy
Pupil	Normal	Small and irregular	Middilated and oval
Response to light	Normal	Poor	Poor
Infection	Conjunctival only	Conjunctival and circumcorneal	Moderate to severe conjunctival and circumcorneal

    C. Mild conjunctivitis associated with an upper respiratory tract infection is usually self-limited and need not be treated.

    D. Purulent conjunctivitis

        1. Cool compresses may decrease the mild discomfort that is occasionally present.

        2. Antimicrobial drops. Continue treatment for one to two days after symptoms have resolved. Instruct patient to use either:

            a. Sodium sulfacetamide 10% (Sodium Sulamyd) ophthalmic solution; instill 1 or 2 drops in the lower conjunctival sac of the affected eye 4 times a day.

            b. Chloramphenicol ophthalmic solution; instill 1 or 2 drops in the lower conjunctival sac of affected eye 4 times a day.

        Note: Aplastic anemia has been reported following the use of chloramphenicol ophthalmic solution.

  VII. Complications

    A. Keratitis and scarring from gonococcus and herpes simplex.

    B. Local allergic reaction to neomycin.

  VIII. Consultation-referral

    A. Any suspicion of uveitis or glaucoma (see Table 4-1).

    B. Cases that might be due to the following:

   1. Gonococcus.

   2. Vaccinia, herpesvirus hominis, herpes zoster.

   3. Foreign body.

   4. Chemical irritants, particularly alkali.

   C. Infants under 1 month of age.

   D. No improvement in 48 hours.

IX. **Follow-up.** Return visit if there is no improvement in 48 hours.

Hordeolum (Stye): Pediatric and Adult

   I. **Definition.** Localized infection of a sebaceous gland along the margin of the eyelid.

  II. **Etiology.** Usually, *Staphylococcus aureus.*

 III. **Clinical features**

   A. Symptoms

   1. Some pain.

   2. No visual disturbances.

   B. Signs

   1. Painful erythematous swelling at the margin of the eyelid.

   2. Sometimes, purulent drainage along the lid margin.

  IV. **Laboratory studies.** None.

   V. **Differential diagnosis**

   A. Infection in a deeper gland, forming a painful swelling that drains on conjunctional surface of the lid.

   B. Tumors or granulomas (rare).

   C. Chronic hordeolum (chalazion).

  VI. **Treatment.** Hot compresses applied for 30 minutes every 3 hours.

 VII. **Complications**

   A. Conjunctivitis.

   B. Cellulitis.

   C. Localized allergic reaction to neomycin.

VIII. **Consultation-referral**

   A. Nonpainful swelling.

   B. Failure to respond within 3 days to treatment.

IX. Follow-up

    A. As necessary for recurrence or failure to heal completely in 10 days.

    B. Return visit in 3 days if there is no improvement.

Cataracts

  I. Definition and etiology. Clouding or opacification of the lens of the eye, which, in 90% of the cases, is associated with aging. More common in diabetics. Rarely associated with hypoparathyroidism, myotonic dystrophy, atopic dermatitis, trauma, drugs such as systemic corticosteroids.

  II. Clinical features

    A. Symptoms. Most commonly, diminution of visual acuity. Less commonly, patients may report an improvement in distant or near vision ("second sight") due to change in refractive error associated with hardening of the lens.

    B. Signs. Opacity of the lens noted when shining pen light directly into pupil or on ophthalmoscopic examination of eye.

  III. Laboratory studies. None.

  IV. Differential diagnosis. Loss of visual acuity due to other causes such as macular degeneration, diabetic retinopathy.

  V. Treatment. The only treatment is surgical removal of the lens. This procedure should be considered only when the cataract causes sufficient visual impairment to reduce the ability of the patient to perform routine daily activities.

  VI. Consultation-referral. As soon as cataracts are readily noted on routine examination, the patient should be referred to an ophthalmologist. Recent improvement in surgical techniques (particularly intraocular lens implantation) suggests that earlier surgical intervention, before severe visual impairment develops, is appropriate.

  VII. Follow-up. By ophthalmologist in 6–12 months.

Disorders of the Ears, Nose, and Throat

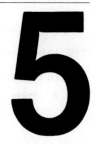

Otitis Externa: Pediatric and Adult

I. **Definition.** Inflammation of the external auditory canal and auricle caused by a variety of infectious agents. May be initiated by trauma from scratching, earplugs, bobby pins, and numerous other foreign objects. Water from swimming or bathing may be absorbed by earwax (cerumen), forming a culture medium for infection.

II. **Etiology**

   A. **Bacteria.** Most commonly *Pseudomonas* Species, *Proteus*, staphylococcus, aureus, and streptococci.

   B. **Fungi**

III. **Clinical features**

   A. **Symptoms**

   1. Pain in ear.

   2. Occasionally, decrease in hearing or a sensation of obstruction in the ear.

   B. **Signs**

   1. Pain is aggravated by movement of the auricle or pressure on the tragus.

   2. The external canal may be partially occluded by edema or discharge.

   3. The external canal is usually tender when examined with an otoscope and is injected or erythematous. Exudate may be seen.

   4. The tympanic membranes may be normal, injected, or covered with flecks of exudate but do not show signs of otitis media; see Acute Purulent Otitis Media (Pediatric and Adult), p. 137, and Serous Otitis Media (Pediatric and Adult), p. 141.

   5. Preauricular or postauricular lymphadenopathy may be present.

      6. There is no swelling or pain over mastoid.

IV. Laboratory studies. None.

V. Differential diagnosis

    A. Otitis media. See Acute Purulent Otitis Media (Pediatric and Adult), p. 138. There may be pus in the external auditory canal in cases of otitis media where perforation of the tympanic membrane has occurred.

    B. Mastoiditis. Swelling and pain over the mastoid area are associated with an abnormal tympanic membrane.

    C. Chronic dermatitides. These usually are not painful but may itch chronically and may be associated with cracking and scaling of the auricle and, in some cases, with discharge. There is usually no pain when the auricle or tragus is moved, unless it is secondarily infected. Types of chronic dermatitides include:

       1. Seborrhea.

       2. Eczema.

       3. Psoriasis.

VI. Treatment

    A. Prevention. Advise patient on the following preventive measures:

       1. Keep fingers and instruments, including cotton swabs, out of ears; the ear canal does *not* need cleaning.

       2. Keep head out of water when taking a bath to avoid filling the ear canals with water and with irritating dirt and soap. (This is a relatively common cause of recurrent otitis externa in children.)

       3. Persistent itching of the external canal warrants medical consultation; do *not* scratch with a foreign object.

    B. Specific therapy. After gently and thoroughly removing debris from the ear canal, give patient the following instructions:

       1. Acetaminophen (Tylenol) for all ages or aspirin for adults for pain; See p. 159 for adult doses and Table 5-5, p. 151 for pediatric doses of Tylenol.

       2. Apply heat to ear by warm compresses, hot water bottle, or heating pad.

       3. Use ear drops. Medication applied to the external ear canal will not be effective unless the canal is sufficiently clear of cerumen and exudate to allow contact with inflamed tissue. Lie with affected ear upward for 5 minutes after drops are instilled.

      a. Cortisporin otic solution (combination of polymyxin B sulfate, neomycin sulfate, and hydrocortisone), 4 drops in the affected ear 4 times a day for 1 week.

      or

      b. Domeboro otic solution (acetic acid, 2%, in aluminum acetate), 4–6 drops in the affected ear 4 times a day for 1 week.

VII. Complications

    A. Severe otitis externa associated with:

      1. Swelling of the canal to complete closure.

      2. Severe pain.

      3. Cellulitis of the canal, auricle, and surrounding tissue.

    B. Local allergic reaction to neomycin.

    C. Patients with diabetes mellitus may have more severe infections.

VIII. Consultation-referral

    A. Severe otitis externa.

      1. Severe pain or fever.

      2. Swelling of external canal sufficient to prevent instillation of drops and requiring a wick.

    B. Cellulitis of ear.

    C. Failure to respond to treatment in 1 week.

    D. More than one recurrence

  IX. Follow-up. Return visit if condition persists after 1 week of treatment.

Acute Purulent Otitis Media: Pediatric and Adult

  I. Definition. Infection in the middle ear, with accumulation of seropurulent or purulent fluid in the middle-ear cavity.

  II. Etiology. The majority of cases are due to bacterial infection. It is not possible clinically to identify those patients with sterile exudate.

  III. Clinical features

    A. Symptoms

      1. Earache.

      2. Symptoms of an upper respiratory infection.

      3. Fever.

4. Decreased hearing.

5. Sometimes, no symptoms.

B. Signs

1. Bulging of any portion of the tympanic membrane with accumulation of exudate in the middle-ear cavity.

2. Disappearance of the malleus (bony landmarks). The short process is often lost first.

3. Perforation of the tympanic membrane, resulting in the presence of exudate in the external canal and distortion of the tympanic membrane. (This must be distinguished from primary otitis externa without otitis media, which is more common in the adult.)

4. Bullae of the tympanic membrane.

5. Decreased or absent movement of the tympanic membrane with insufflation.

Note: Injection or erythema of the tympanic membrane and disappearance or distortion of the light reflex may accompany these signs but are not alone sufficient to diagnose acute purulent otitis media.

IV. Laboratory studies. None.

V. Differential diagnosis

A. Erythema of the tympanic membrane associated with an upper respiratory tract infection.

B. Serous otitis media.

C. Otitis externa.

VI. Treatment. Ask whether patient is allergic to the medication chosen.

A. Patients under 18 years of age. Be sure infant is not being fed in the supine position, since this may predispose to otitis media.

1. Amoxicillin:

a. Patients weighing 6–10 kg (13–22 lb) (see Table 5-1 for dosage).

b. Patients weighing over 10 kg (22 lb) (see Table 5-2 for dosage).

2. If patient is allergic to penicillin derivatives, or if there is reason to suspect that the causative organism is an ampicillin- or amoxicillin-resistant strain of *Hemophilus influenzae*, treat with erythromycin and sulfisoxazole combination (Pediazole); see Table 5-3, p. 139, for dosage.

Table 5-1. Oral pediatric dosage of amoxicillin suspension (125 mg per 5 ml) for treatment of acute purulent otitis media

Body weight	Dose	Frequency
6–8 kg (13–18 kg)	100 mg (4 ml)	Every 8 hours for 10 days
8–10 kg (18–22 lb)	125 mg (5 ml)	

Table 5-2. Oral pediatric dosage of amoxicillin suspension (250 mg per 5 ml)

Body weight	Dose	Frequency
10–12 kg (22–26 lb)	150 mg (3 ml)	
12–15 kg (26–33 lb)	200 mg (4 ml)	Every 8 hours for 10 days
Over 15 kg (over 33 lb)	250 mg[a] (5 ml)	

[a]Patients weighing more than 15 kg (over 33 lb) who are able to safely swallow capsules may be given amoxicillin capsules, 250 mg 3 times a day for 10 days, or ampicillin, 250 mg 4 times a day for 10 days.

Table 5-3. Oral dosage of erythromycin ethylsuccinate (200 mg per 5 ml) and sulfisoxazole acetyl (600 mg per 5 ml) suspension combination (pediazole)

Body weight	Dose	Frequency
6–9 kg (13–20 lb)	2 ml	
9–12 kg (20–26 lb)	3 ml	
12–16 kg (26–35 lb)	4 ml	
16–20 kg (35–44 lb)	5 ml	
20–24 kg (44–53 lb)	6 ml	4 times a day for 10 days
24–28 kg (53–62 lb)	7 ml	
28–32 kg (62–70 lb)	8 ml	
Over 32 kg (over 70 lb)	10 ml	

B. Patients over 18 years of age

1. Amoxicillin capsules, 250 mg 3 times a day for 10 days.

   or

2. If patient is allergic to penicillin derivatives, treat with 80 mg trimethoprim, 400 mg sulfamethoxazole tablets, two tablets 2 times a day for 10 days.

VII. Complications

A. Chronic serous otitis media (persistent middle ear effusion).

B. Persistent purulent otitis media.

C. Mastoiditis.

D. Chronic otitis media with perforation of the tympanic membrane.

E. Extension into the central nervous system, leading to meningitis or brain abscess.

F. Cholesteatoma formation associated with chronic otitis media and marginal or pars flaccida perforation.

VIII. Consultation-referral

A. Infants under 3 months of age.

B. Severe pain.

C. Failure to improve symptomatically in 48 hours.

D. Signs of meningitis, such as:

1. Lethargy.

2. Extreme irritability.

3. Bulging fontanel.

4. Stiff neck.

E. Persistent purulent otitis media, despite adequate course of antibiotics.

F. More than two episodes of purulent otitis media:

1. Child—in 1 year.

2. Adult—over any period of time.

G. Suspicion of mastoiditis (pain, tenderness, or edema in the postauricular area in older children and adults).

H. Chronic otitis media with persistent intermittent drainage through perforation of the tympanic membrane.

IX. Follow-up. Examination in 3 weeks.

Serous Otitis Media: Pediatric and Adult

  I. **Definition.** Accumulation of a bacteriologically sterile, nonpurulent effusion in the middle-ear cavity.

 II. **Etiology**

   A. Eustachian tube obstruction with subsequent formation of an effusion in the middle-ear cavity. The causes of eustachian tube obstruction include:

   1. Enlarged adenoids.

   2. Upper respiratory tract infection with mucosal edema.

   3. Allergic rhinitis with mucosal edema.

   4. Cleft palate.

   5. Deviated nasal septum.

   6. Nasopharyngeal tumor in adults.

   B. A complication of purulent otitis media.

   C. Possibly, active secretion by the mucosa of the middle-ear cavity in an allergic patient.

III. **Clinical features**

   A. Symptoms

   1. Hearing loss.

   2. Feeling of fullness in the ear.

   3. Snapping sensation when swallowing, yawning, or blowing the nose.

   4. Symptoms associated with the disorders listed in **II.A** (e.g., chronic snoring associated with enlarged adenoids).

   5. Occasionally, no symptoms, especially if chronic.

   B. Signs

   1. Clear or transparent yellowish fluid (early) or bluish gray fluid (longstanding), with or without air bubbles behind the tympanic membrane associated with

      a. Retraction of the tympanic membrane.

      b. Prominence of the malleus, especially the short process, with an abnormally horizontal handle of the malleus drawn inward.

      c. Decreased or absent movement of the tympanic membrane with insufflation. Occasionally, only outward movement with negative pressure is seen.

Note: Injection or erythema of the tympanic membrane and disappearance or distortion of the light reflex, as seen in an upper respiratory tract infection or allergic rhinitis, may accompany these signs but are not alone sufficient to diagnose serous otitis media.

2. Signs associated with the disorders listed in **II.A** (e.g., mouth breathing associated with enlarged adenoids).

3. Decreased hearing.

IV. Laboratory studies. None.

V. Differential diagnosis

A. Acute purulent otitis media.

B. Chronic otitis media.

C. Retraction or erythema, or both, of the tympanic membrane without serous effusion, as seen in an upper respiratory tract infection or allergic rhinitis.

D. Normal retracted appearance of the tympanic membrane of very young infant.

E. Symptoms of eustachian tube obstruction alone, with a normal tympanic membrane.

F. Hearing loss due to other causes.

G. Ménière's disease.

VI. Treatment

A. Children under 12 years of age

1. Be sure infant is not being fed in the supine position, which may predispose to otitis media.

2. No therapy. Serous otitis media resolves spontaneously in most patients.

3. Return appointment in 6 weeks. If middle-ear effusion is still present at that time, patient should be referred.

B. Adults and children over 12 years of age

1. No therapy if asymptomatic or if symptoms are minimal. Serous otitis media resolves spontaneously in almost all patients in this age group.

2. If patient is symptomatic or if middle ear effusion is still present after 3 weeks, prescribe topical decongestant.

a. Xylometazoline HCl (Otrivin) 0.1% nasal solution, 2 or 3 drops in each nostril every 8 hours.

or

b. Xylometazoline HCl (Otrivin) 0.1% nasal spray, 1 spray followed in 5–10 minutes by a second spray; repeat sequence every 8 hours.

3. If condition is not resolved after 2 weeks of therapy outlined in **2**, refer patient.

VII. Complications

A. Chronic serous otitis media (persistent middle-ear effusion) with increased risk of

1. Decreased hearing, which can contribute to:

a. Learning difficulties in school.

b. Defective speech development.

2. Adhesive otitis media, with permanent conductive hearing loss.

B. Acute purulent otitis media.

C. Cholesteatoma from chronic severe retraction of pars flaccida.

VIII. Consultation-referral

A. Children under 12 years of age

1. Failure to resolve after 3 weeks.

2. More than two episodes in 1 year.

B. Adults and children over 12 years of age

1. Failure to resolve after 2 weeks of therapy outlined in **VI.B.2**.

2. More than two episodes in 1 year.

IX. Follow-up

A. See **VI.A** or **B**.

B. To avoid complications, always follow patients until resolution occurs.

Epistaxis: Pediatric and Adult

I. **Definition.** The spontaneous discharge of blood from the nares.

II. **Etiology**

A. Spontaneous rupture of a blood vessel in the nose (usually the anterior septum), occurring most frequently in children and in the elderly.

B. Higher incidence in winter, when heating causes drying and cracking of nasal mucosa.

C. Trauma from a direct blow to the nose.

D. Picking of dry, crusted nostrils.

E. Rarely, hypertension.

F. Rarely, a bleeding disorder.

III. Clinical features

A. Symptoms. Usually, none, other than the awareness of blood dripping down the posterior nasopharynx as well as external bleeding.

B. Signs

1. Bleeding from the nares and down the posterior nasopharynx.

2. Localized bleeding point (may or may not be seen in the anterior nasal septum).

3. Usually, normal blood pressure.

4. Usually, no orthostatic fall in blood pressure.

5. Usually, no evidence of bleeding or clotting disorder (e.g., bruises, petechiae).

IV. Laboratory studies

A. Generally, none.

B. Hematocrit, if history indicates significant bleeding.

V. Differential diagnosis. None.

VI. Treatment

A. Acute bleeding

1. Keep the patient in an erect sitting position with head tilted forward to prevent blood from going down the posterior nasopharynx.

2. To decrease venous pressure, try to keep children from crying.

3. With thumb and forefinger, apply continuous external compression on both sides of the nose for 15 minutes.

B. Prevention

1. Discourage picking of the nose.

2. Advise patient to increase the humidity in the home, especially in sleeping areas, by means of a humidifier or pot of water on a heater.

3. Tell patient to rub petrolatum over the nasal septum twice a day when dry or crusted.

VII. Complications. Anemia, if bleeding is excessive or frequent.

VIII. Consultation-referral

A. Bleeding not controlled by 15 minutes of compression.

B. Evidence of massive bleeding.

C. Recurrent bleeding within first hour.

D. Second episode within a week.

E. Bleeding from the posterior nasopharynx (usually cannot be controlled by the measures described in **VI.A.**)

IX. Follow-up. As needed for recurrent episodes.

Allergic Rhinitis: Pediatric and Adult

I. Definition. An allergic disease affecting the nasal mucosa and often the conjunctiva. It may be seasonal or perennial (nonseasonal).

II. Etiology

A. **Seasonal**

1. Pollens that depend on wind for cross-pollination. In the eastern United States, the following are the most common causes (pollination time may vary by several months depending on location):

a. Ragweed, August–October.

b. Grasses, May–July.

c. Trees, April–July.

d. Combinations of **a, b,** and **c.**

B. **Perennial**

1. House dust.

2. Feathers.

3. Mold spores.

4. Animal dander.

5. Foods. There is disagreement about the role of food in causing isolated allergic rhinitis. Most authorities believe that if foods are causative, other signs of hypersensitivity occur with allergic rhinitis (e.g., urticaria, asthma, gastrointestinal symptoms).

C. Perennial with seasonal exacerbations

D. Aggravating factors

1. Tobacco smoke.

2. Air pollutants.

3. Sudden temperature changes.

III. Clinical features

A. Symptoms. Onset is usually in childhood and young adulthood, with symptoms decreasing with age. A family history of allergic diseases is common. Symptoms of seasonal allergic rhinitis tend to occur the same time each year and are frequently more severe than those of the perennial form.

1. Sneezing.

2. Nasal itching.

3. Watery rhinorrhea.

4. Nasal stuffiness.

5. Occasionally, other symptoms including:

   a. Itching of the eyes, palate, and throat.

   b. Snoring and sniffing.

   c. Increased tearing and photophobia.

   d. Nonproductive cough from irritation of posterior pharyngeal secretions.

   e. Fatigue, irritability, anorexia.

B. Signs

1. Clear, thin nasal discharge.

2. Pale, edematous nasal mucosa.

3. Enlarged nasal turbinates.

4. "Allergic salute," that is, rubbing of the nose upward and outward (seen especially in children).

5. Mouth-breathing.

6. Conjunctival injection and edema. Occasionally granular, erythematous conjunctivae and swollen eyelids, with extra lines and dark semicircles (allergic "shiners") under the eyes.

7. Allergic facies with perennial allergic rhinitis:

   a. Mouth-breathing.

   b. Prominent maxilla, high arched palate.

    c. Dull expression.

    d. Broad midsection of nose, with horizontal crease across lower portion.

IV. Laboratory studies. Wright's or Hansel's stain of smear of nasal secretions may reveal eosinophils, but usually is not needed to make a diagnosis.

V. Differential diagnosis

  A. Seasonal

    1. Upper respiratory tract infection.

    2. Infectious conjunctivitis.

  B. Perennial

    1. Recurrent upper respiratory tract infections.

    2. Vasomotor rhinitis (of unknown cause, noninfectious, nonseasonal, and nonallergic).

    3. Deviated nasal septum.

    4. Side effect of medications, such as reserpine and vasoconstricting nose drops.

    5. Chronic sinusitis.

VI. Treatment

  A. Identification and avoidance of the offending antigen. Advise patient on the following measures *if appropriate* for that individual:

    1. Seasonal

      a. Avoid areas of heavy concentration of ragweed, trees, or grass during pollinating seasons.

      b. Sleep with bedroom windows closed during the appropriate pollinating season.

      c. Use an air conditioner with an electrostatic precipitating filter to avoid pollen.

    2. Perennial

      a. Create a dust-free bedroom (patients who must do their own cleaning should use a mouth-and-nose mask):

        (1) Remove everything from the room, including floor coverings, curtains, drapes, and closet contents.

        (2) Clean the room thoroughly—walls, woodwork, ceiling, floor, and closet. Wax the floor.

        (3) Scrub the bed frame and metal springs.

(4) Cover the mattress, box spring, and pillows with plastic dustproof covers.

(5) Make sure the room contains a minimum of furniture, washable rugs, and curtains. Avoid bed pads, heavy rugs, drapes, upholstered furniture, toys, and knickknacks.

(6) Clean the room at least once a week using a vacuum cleaner, damp cloth, or oil mop. Do not use a broom or duster.

(7) Keep bedroom windows and doors closed. If hot-air heating is used, cover vents with coarse muslin and change frequently. Change furnace air filter frequently.

b. Vaccum stuffed furniture and rugs frquently.

c. Keep pets (dogs, cats) away from the bedroom.

d. Avoid damp and dusty places (attics, basements, closets, storerooms).

e. Avoid stuffed toys, if patient is dust-sensitive.

f. Use an air conditioner with an electrostatic precipitating filter to avoid dust.

B. Antihistamine. Use chlorpheniramine (Chlor-Trimeton); see Table 3-4, p. 126, for dosage.

Note: The goal of therapy is to achieve symptomatic relief with a minimum of side effects (e.g., drowsiness, nervousness, dry mouth). Therefore, manipulation of dosage within the prescribed ranges may be necessary. Medication should be taken for several days to weeks to a time during symptomatic periods; since antihistamines do not antagonize released histamine but only prevent further release, intermittent single-dose usage will not be as effective in controlling symptoms.

VII. Complications

A. Eustachian tube obstruction causing serous otitis media.

B. Sinus orifice obstruction causing sinusitis.

C. Nasal or sinus polyps from long-standing perennial allergic rhinitis.

D. Dental malocclusion problems from maxillary deformity associated with chronic nasal obstruction.

E. Drowsiness from antihistamine therapy.

VIII. Consultation-referral

A. Failure to rspond to treatment.

B. Consideration for immunotherapy (hyposensitization):

1. Severe or prolonged periods of symptoms not controlled by treatment measures described above.

2. Inability to tolerate antihistamines; symptoms that are more than mild.

3. Patients requiring almost daily medication for perennial allergic rhinitis.

IX. **Follow-up.** Return visit in 1 week, and periodically as needed.

Pharyngitis (Sore Throat): Pediatric and Adult

I. **Definition.** Inflammation of the pharynx or tonsils, or both.

II. **Etiology**

A. Usually nonbacterial (presumed to be viral).

B. Group A beta-hemolytic streptococci.

C. Much less commonly, *Mycoplasma pneumoniae.*

D. Unusual in the United States, Corynebacterium diphtheriae.

E. Unusual, Neisseria meningitides and gonorrhoeae.

F. Possibly a cause, Chlamydia trachomatis.

III. **Clinical features.** It is *not* possible to determine the etiology of pharyngitis by clinical features alone. Although Table 5-4 may be helpful, a throat culture is needed to definitely establish whether or not pharyngitis is due to group A beta-hemolytic streptococci. Streptococcal pharyngitis is unusual under 3 years of age.

IV. **Laboratory studies**

A. Throat culture of patient for group A beta-hemolytic streptococci.

B. Throat culture of all *symptomatic* family and close contacts of patient with streptococcal pharyngitis.

C. Throat culture of *all* family and close contacts of patient with streptococcal pharyngitis under the following conditions:

1. The patient or one of the contacts has a history of rheumatic fever.

or

2. There is an outbreak of rheumatic fever or poststreptococcal glomerulonephritis in the community.

D. White blood cell and differential counts and heterophile antibody determination in suspected cases of infectious mononucleosis; see Chapter 16, Infectious Mononucleosis (Pediatric and Adult), pp. 347–348.

Table 5-4. Findings in pharyngitis suggestive of streptococcal etiology

Clinical feature	Very suggestive	Moderately suggestive	Questionably suggestive	Unusual
Tender enlarged anterior cervical lymph nodes	All ages			
Household contact	All ages			
Scarletina from rash	School age Adults			Infants
Excoriated nares	Infants			School age Adults
Tonsillar exudate	Adults	School age	Infants	
High fever		All ages		
Occurrence during winter and spring		All ages		
Acute onset		School age Adults		Infants
Sore throat		School age Adults		Infants
Abdominal pain		Infants School age		Adults
Rhinorrhea		Infants		School age Adults
Red throat			All ages	
Hoarseness				All ages
Cough				All ages

Source: Modified from L. A. Wannamaker, *Am. J. Dis. Child.* 124:357, 1972.

V. Differential diagnosis

   A. Infectious mononucleosis.

   B. Influenza.

   C. Stomatitis (e.g., herpetic).

VI. Treatment

A. General measures for pharyngitis of any etiology

   1. Acetaminophen (Tylenol) for all ages or aspirin for adults for high fever; see p. 159 for adult doses and Table 5-5, p. 151 for pediatric doses of Tylenol.

   2. Warm saline gargle for older children and adults.

   3. Increased fluid intake.

Table 5-5. Oral pediatric dosage of acetaminophen (Tylenol)

Age	Dose		Frequency
	Drops (60 mg/0.6 ml)	Elixir (120 mg/5 ml)	
3 months–1 year	0.6 ml *or*	2.5 ml	
1–3 years	0.6–1.2 ml *or*	2.5–5.0 ml	As often as
3–6 years	1.2 ml *or*	5.0 ml	every 6 hours
Over 6 years*	· · ·	10.0 ml	

*Alternative is one-half to one tablet (325 mg per tablet) 3 or 4 times daily.

B. Antibiotics for streptococcal pharyngitis. Ask whether patient is allergic to penicillin.

Note: Tetracyclines and sulfonamides should not be used for the treatment of streptococcal pharyngitis.

1. Benzathine penicillin G (Bicillin). (Mixtures containing penicillin are acceptable; however, the dosage of benzathine pencillin G should *not* be decreased from that listed below.)

   a. Patients weighing less than 25 kg (55 lb): One IM injection of 600,000 units.

   b. Patients weighing more than 25 kg (55 lb): One IM injection of 1,200,000 units.

   Note: Patients should be observed by health care providers for at least 20 minutes after receiving injections.

   or

2. **Oral penicillin.** This method of therapy depends on the cooperation of the patient for 10 days. Because many patients do not understand the need for taking medication for the full 10 days, IM benzathine penicillin G is usually the method of choice. If oral penicillin is selected, however, specific counseling outlining the need for the 10 full days of therapy to eradicate the infection and prevent rheumatic fever should be stressed. Dosage is penicillin V, 250 mg 3 times a day for 10 days.

   or

3. **If patient is allergic to penicillin,** use

   a. Erythromycin suspension (see Table 3-3, p. 113, for dosage).

   or

   b. If patient is over 25 kg (55 lb), erythromycin tablets (250 mg per tablet) in a dosage of 500 mg (2 tablets) twice a day for 10 days taken 1 hour before meals.

Note: If abdominal discomfort develops, divide dose in half and give 4 times a day.

VII. Complications of streptococcal pharyngitis

A. Rheumatic fever.

B. Cervical lymphadenitis, particularly in infants.

C. Otitis media, particularly in children.

D. Peritonsillar abscess in older children and adults.

E. Retropharyngeal abscess in younger children.

F. Sinusitis.

G. Acute glomerulonephritis.

VIII. Consultation-referral

A. Cervical adenitis of 3 cm in diameter or greater.

B. Peritonsillar abscess. Consider when the following are present:

1. Asymmetrical swelling of tonsils, tonsillar fossae, and overlying soft palate. Uvula shifted to opposite side.

2. Fever persisting 4 days after treatment for streptococcal pharyngitis was started.

3. Trismus, difficulty in swallowing, and feeling of fullness in throat.

4. Extreme enlargement of tonsils.

C. Prolonged toxic course

D. Retropharyngeal abscess. Consider in infant when the following are present:

1. Difficulty in swallowing.

2. Persistent high fever.

3. Hyperextended head, with difficulty in breathing.

4. Forward bulge in the posterior pharyngeal wall.

E. Membrane on pharynx suggesting diphtheria.

IX. Follow-up. Throat cultures of the patient with streptococcal pharyngitis and family members and close contacts are generally *not* indicated unless:

A. Someone is symptomatic.

B. The patient or a contact has a history of rheumatic fever.

C. There is an outbreak of rheumatic fever or poststreptococcal glomerulonephritis in the community.

Note: If someone has a positive repeat culture for Group A beta-hemolytic streptococci, treat only one more time and do *not* reculture after treatment.

Oral Candidiasis (Thrush): Pediatric

I. **Definition.** Superficial fungal infection of the oral cavity in infants.

II. **Etiology.** The causative organism is *Candida albicans,* which is usually acquired from the following sources:

  A. Mother's vagina during birth.

  B. Other infants, by contamination of caretaker's hands or objects shared by babies.

  C. Adult with vaginal candidiasis, through contamination of her hands.

  D. Patient's own candidal diaper dermatitis.

  E. Oral broad-spectrum antibiotic therapy (e.g., ampicillin), as a side effect.

III. **Clinical features**

  A. Symptoms

  1. Often none.

  2. With extensive involvement, pain during feeding and swallowing.

  B. Signs

  1. White, irregularly shaped plaques appear on the buccal mucosa, lips, palate, and gums. They may produce a confluent white coating on the tongue.

  2. Lesions are removable, leaving an inflamed base.

  3. The patient may have candidal diaper dermatitis (moist, red, occasionally scaling rash with a sharp border and satellite red papules or pustules).

IV. **Laboratory studies.** Potassium hydroxide preparation of scrapings of lesions reveals budding yeast with or without hyphae. This study usually is not needed when typical lesions are present.

V. **Differential diagnosis.** Milk or food particles remaining in the mouth of the patient.

VI. **Treatment.** Advise parent on the following measures:

A. **Control of source of infection**

1. Wash hands thoroughly between handling of different infants in newborn nursery and before handling any baby.

2. Do not have infants share clothing, pacifiers, or nipples.

3. Examine and treat contact with vaginitis.

4. Treat candidal diaper dermatitis (see Chapter 3, Diaper Dermatitis, **VI.D,** p. 100).

B. **Oral antifungal therapy.** Use nystatin (Mycostatin) oral suspension (100,000 units per milliliter) in a dosage of 2 ml orally 4 times a day for 1 week (1 ml in each side of mouth, not in back of throat, so that medication is in contact with the lesions for as long as possible). It may help to rub a portion of the dose on the lesions with a cotton swab. This oral antifungal treatment may be repeated for another week if there is not marked improvement.

VII. **Complications**

A. Feeding problems due to pain.

B. Candidal diaper dermatitis or perioral dermatitis.

C. Spread of infection to other infants in nursery or home.

VIII. **Consultation-referral**

A. Failure to respond to 2 weeks of therapy.

B. Failure to thrive.

IX. **Follow-up.** Return visit in 1 week if the infection is not markedly improved.

Bacterial Sinusitis: Adult

I. **Definition.** Inflammation of the mucous membrane lining of the paranasal sinuses due to bacterial infection, causing obstruction of normal sinus discharge. In chronic recurrent disease, allergens or irritants such as smoke may initiate symptoms.

II. **Etiology**

A. **Most common**

1. Hemophilus influenza.

2. Streptococcus pneumonia.

3. Various anaerobes.

B. **Less common**

  1. Neisseria species.

  2. Beta-hemolytic streptococci.

  3. Staphylococcus aureus.

  4. Escherichia coli.

III. Clinical features

A. Symptoms

  1. Mucopurulent nasal discharge and persistent postnasal drip.

  2. Choking cough at night, often appearing after a recent upper respiratory tract infection.

  3. General malaise.

  4. An ache or pressure behind the eyes.

  5. Toothache-like pain.

  6. Headache (often worse at night and early morning).

B. Signs

  1. Yellow mucopurulent nasal discharge.

  2. Tenderness over the involved sinus.

  3. Edematous, hyperemic inferior turbinates.

  4. Usually, fever (101°F or higher).

  5. Failure of sinus to transilluminate.

IV. Laboratory and other studies

  A. X-ray (only on physician's orders).

  B. Nasopharyngeal cultures correlate poorly with cultures obtained by sinus aspiration and are therefore not indicated.

V. Differential diagnosis

  A. Nonbacterial sinusitis.

  B. Undifferentiated upper respiratory tract infection.

  C. Persistent rhinitis due to allergy.

VI. Treatment

A. Nasal congestion and drainage. Advise patient on the following measures:

  1. Keep head raised when lying down.

  2. Use a topical decongestant:

    a. Xylometazoline HCl (Otrivin) 0.1% nasal solution, 2 or 3 drops in each nostril every 8 hours for a maximum of 2 weeks.

or

b. Xylometazoline HCl (Otrivin) 0.1% nasal spray, 1 spray followed in 5–10 minutes by a second spray; repeat sequence every 8 hours for a maximum of 2 weeks.

and/or

3. Start oral therapy:

a. Pseudoephedrine HCl (Sudafed) tablets (60 mg per tablet), 1 tablet 3 or 4 times a day for a maximum of 2 weeks.

or

b. Phenylpropanolamine HCl (Propadrine) tablets (50 mg per table), 1 tablet 3 or 4 times a day for a maximum of 2 weeks.

or

c. Triprolidine HCl and pseudoephedrine HCl (Actifed) tablets, 1 tablet 3 times a day for a maximum of 2 weeks.

B. Fever or pain. Have patient take aspirin (325 mg per tablet), 2 tablets orally every 4–6 hours.

C. Infection. Patient can take antibiotics, but prescribe *only* after telephone consultation with physician.

1. Ampicillin, 500 mg orally 4 times a day for 10 days if not allergic to penicillin.

or

2. Erythromycin, 250 mg orally 4 times a day for 10 days if allergic to penicillin.

VII. Complications. Complications are infrequent but serious.

A. Abscess.

B. Osteomyelitis.

C. Spread to the central nervous system.

VIII. Consultation-referral

A. All patients with acute frontal sinusitis.

B. All acutely and severely ill patients.

C. Chronic or recurrent illness.

D. Any indication of involvement of the orbit or central nervous system.

IX. Follow-up. Have patient call in 2-3 days if there is no improvement.

Nonbacterial Sinusitis: Adult

I. **Definition.** Inflammation of the mucous membrane lining the paranasal sinuses due to viral, allergic, vasomotor, or other nonbacterial causes, producing obstruction of normal sinus discharge.

II. **Etiology**

   A. Numerous viruses, pollens, and other allergens.

   B. Vasomotor instability secondary to cold or emotional factors, or both.

III. **Clinical features**

   A. **Symptoms**

   1. Clear, nonpurulent nasal discharge.

   2. Nocturnal postnasal drip with resultant cough.

   3. Pain in the area of the involved sinuses that is usually appreciated as a sensation of pressure or fullness.

   4. Minimal or no generalized symptoms, such as malaise or myalgia.

   5. Headache.

   6. Simulation of a toothache in some cases of maxillary sinusitis.

   B. **Signs**

   1. Clear nasal discharge.

   2. Edema and hyperemia of the nasal mucosa.

   3. Tenderness over the involved sinus.

   4. No erythema of the area over the involved sinus.

   5. No fever, or temperature less than 101°F.

IV. **Laboratory studies.** None.

V. **Differential diagnosis**

   A. Bacterial sinusitis.

   B. Uncomplicated upper respiratory tract infection.

   C. Allergic rhinitis.

   D. Dental abscess.

VI. **Treatment.** Advise patient on the following measures:

   A. **Nasal congestion.** In sinusitis alone and in sinusitis associated with viral upper respiratory infection, the use of decongestants or antihistamines, or both, is usually sufficient to decrease edema and discomfort. For treatment measures, see Bacterial Sinusitis (Adult), **VI.A,** pp. 155–156.

B. Pain. Aspirin (325 mg per tablet), 2 tablets every 4–6 hours as needed.

VII. **Complications.** Bacterial sinusitis.

VIII. **Consultation-referral.** Chronic or recurrent illness.

IX. **Follow-up.** Telephone call in 2–3 days if no improvement.

Upper Respiratory Tract Infection (Common Cold): Pediatric and Adult

I. **Definition.** An acute infection of the upper respiratory tract lasting several days.

II. **Etiology.** Numerous viruses.

III. **Clinical features**

A. **Symptoms**

1. General malaise.

2. Nasal stuffiness, nasal discharge, sneezing, cough.

3. Mild sore throat.

4. Water eyes.

5. Decreased appetite, particularly in infants.

B. **Signs**

1. Erythematous, edematous nasal mucosa, with clear, thin nasal discharge initially. The discharge may become mucoid or purulent as the illness resolves.

2. Mildly erythematous pharynx.

3. Mild conjunctivitis.

4. Sometimes, fever. It is usually of low grade, but may be elevated in infants.

5. Erythematous tympanic membranes in infants.

IV. **Laboratory studies**

A. Usually, none.

B. Nasal culture for group A beta-hemolytic streptococci if nasal discharge persists for more than 2 weeks in an infant under 2 years of age and is associated with anorexia, fever, cervical lymphadenopathy, or, especially, excoriation and crusting around the nostrils.

Table 5-6. Pediatric dosage of 0.05% xylometazoline (Otrivin) nasal solution

Age	Dose (in each nostril)	Frequency
6 months–2 years	2 drops	Every 8 hours while awake as needed[a]
2–12 years	3 drops	Every 8 hours while awake as needed[a]

[a]Do not use for more than 3 days.

V. Differential diagnosis

A. Allergic rhinitis.

B. Foreign body, particularly if nasal discharge is unilateral and malodorous, purulent, or bloody.

VI. Treatment

A. Increased oral fluid intake

B. Aspiration of nasal secretions with rubber suction bulb in infants, particularly before feedings.

C. Antipyretics and analgesics

1. Children. Acetaminophen (Tylenol) as needed for high fever (see Table 5-5, p. 151, for dosage).

2. Adults

a. Acetaminophen (325 mg per tablet), 1 or 2 tablets as often as every 6 hours as needed.

or

b. Aspirin (325 mg per tablet), 1 or 2 tablets as often as every 4 hours as needed.

D. Topical decongestant for nasal stuffiness or discharge.

1. Children under 12 years of age.

Note: The nasal stuffiness and discharge of the common cold are self-limiting, and most patients do not need medication. When symptoms are causing distress or poor feeding and are not controlled by nasal bulb-syringe aspiration in infants, then medication may be helpful. Use xylometazoline HCl (Otrivin) 0.05% nasal solution (see Table 5-6 for dosage).

2. Adults and children over 12 years of age

a. Xylometazoline HCl (Otrivin) 0.1% nasal solution, 2 or 3 drops in each nostril every 8 hours as needed. Do not use for more than 3 days.

or

b. Xylometazoline HCl (Otrivin) 0.1% nasal spray, 1 spray followed by a second spray in 5–10 minutes; repeat sequence every 8 hours as needed. Do not use for more than 3 days.

and/or

c. Oral decongestant-antihistamine combination, such as triprolidine HCl and pseudoephedrine HCl (Actifed) tablets, 1 tablet 3 times a day.

VII. Complications

A. Serous or purulent otitis media, particularly in infants and young children.

B. Sinusitis.

C. Lower respiratory tract infection.

VIII. Consultation-referral. Only if indicated for a complication.

IX. Follow-up. As needed.

Disorders of the Lower Respiratory System

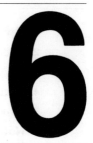

Acute Laryngotracheobronchitis (Viral Croup): Pediatric

I. **Definition.** Inflammation of the larynx, often extending to the subglottis, trachea, and bronchi, characterized by hoarseness, barking cough, and inspiratory stridor, usually occurring between ages 6 months and 5 years.

II. **Etiology.** Myxoviruses (parainfluenza types 1, 2, and 3, and influenza virus types A and B).

III. **Clinical features**

   A. **Symptoms**

   1. Barking cough.

   2. Inspiratory stridor.

   3. Hoarseness.

   4. Labored breathing.

   5. Symptoms usually occur or become worse at night.

   6. Common cold symptoms usually precede onset.

   B. **Signs**

   1. Inspiratory stridor.

   2. Barking cough.

   3. Hoarseness.

   4. Labored breathing with respiratory distress.

   5. Low-grade or absent fever.

IV. **Diagnostic studies.** Chest and lateral neck x-ray films only after consultation, but usually these are not needed.

V. **Differential diagnosis**

   A. Acute epiglottitis caused by *Hemophilus influenzae* type B and suggested by the following:

    1. Fever over 101°F rectally.

    2. Sudden onset, with rapid progression.

    3. Severe respiratory distress.

    4. Toxicity, agitation, or prostration.

    5. Drooling, with sore throat or difficulty in swallowing, or both.

    Note: Do *not* attempt to look at the epiglottis or upset the patient. This can lead to complete obstruction.

  B. Congenital laryngeal stridor in infant.

  C. Aspirated foreign body.

  D. Diphtheria.

VI. Treatment. Advise parent on these measures:

  A. Change environmental air to increase humidity:

    1. Let patient breath outside air when symptoms increase (usually at night).

    2. Place patient in a steam-filled room (e.g., bathroom where hot water had been running).

  B. Increase fluid intake.

VII. Complications

  A. Airway obstruction.

  B. Severe tracheobronchitis.

  C. Pneumonia.

VIII. Consultation-referral

  A. Signs of epiglottitis. *Refer immediately—this is an emergency.*

  B. Respiratory distress.

IX. Follow-up. Return visit if there is an increase in symptoms.

Acute Tracheobronchitis: Pediatric

  I. Definition. Acute inflammation of the respiratory epithelium of the trachea and bronchi without involvement of the alveoli or supporting lung tissue.

  II. Etiology

    A. A viral etiology is most common, particularly in young children. Any of the viral respiratory pathogens may be responsible, but the myxoviruses (the parainfluenza viruses and influenza virus types A and B) are most common.

B. *Mycoplasma pneumoniae* is a common cause in school-age children and adolescents.

III. Clinical features

A. Symptoms

1. Cough (persistent, dry, and worse at night).

2. Sometimes, mild tachypnea.

3. Restlessness and irritability associated with cough.

4. Sometimes, preceding or accompanying symptoms of upper respiratory tract infection.

5. Sometimes, systemic symptoms, including myalgia, headache, anorexia, and lethargy, particularly with influenza viruses.

B. Signs

1. Rhonchi.

2. High-pitched inspiratory or expiratory wheezing that improves with coughing.

3. Fever—usually absent or of low grade; sometimes high, particularly with influenza viruses.

4. Often preceded or accompanied by signs of upper respiratory tract infection.

IV. Diagnostic studies. Chest x-ray only after consultation. Usually x-ray not needed.

V. Differential diagnosis

A. Uncomplicated upper respiratory tract infection.

B. Pneumonia.

C. Bronchial asthma.

D. Viral croup (laryngotracheobronchitis).

E. Aspirated irritants, particularly hydrocarbons.

F. Aspirated foreign body.

G. Tuberculosis and other chronic pulmonary diseases.

H. Congestive heart failure.

VI. Treatment

A. **Prevention.** Influenza virus vaccine (subvirion or split-virus preparations) is strongly recommended for children over 6 months of age with chronic cardiorespiratory diseases or with compromised immune systems.

B. **Therapy**

1. Increased oral fluid intake.

2. Adequate environmental humidity.

3. Soothing preparations, such as lemon juice mixed with sugar.

4. No antibiotics, as most cases are of viral origin.

5. Tuberculin skin test:

   a. If there has not been one in a year.

   b. If there is a question of exposure to tuberculosis.

   c. If symptoms persist.

6. Acetaminophen (Tylenol) for fever (see Table 5-5, p. 151, for dosage).

   Note: Aspirin should *not* be used if influenza is suspected, because there is evidence that it may be associated with the development of Reye's syndrome in patients with influenza or chickenpox.

7. Avoid use of cough medications, particularly those which contain cough suppressants, in children.

VII. Complications

A. Usually, none.

B. Rarely, bacterial pneumonia.

VIII. Consultation-referral

A. Respiratory distress.

B. Evidence of systemic toxicity.

C. More than two episodes in a year.

D. Symptoms lasting more than 3 weeks.

E. Suspicion of aspiration.

IX. Follow-up

A. Clinic visit if no improvement in 7 days.

B. Children with chronic cardiorespiratory disease should be seen again in 2–3 days.

C. Return visit if symptoms of respiratory distress develop.

Acute Lower Respiratory Tract Infections (Adult)*
(Acute Bronchitis)

I. **Definition.** An infectious inflammatory disease primarily of the bronchi characterized by one or more of these: hyperemia of the bronchial mucosa, increased production of mucus, an inflammatory exudate of mucus and white blood cells. There may be some inflammatory involvement of the alveolar spaces.*

II. **Etiology.** Viruses are the most common cause. Other common agents are the bacteria *Streptococcus pneumoniae* and *Hemophilus influenzae,* and *Mycoplasma pneumoniae.* Much less commonly, a wide spectrum of infectious agents can produce acute bronchitis (e.g., Legionella, pertussis).

*Note: Acute lower respiratory tract infections in adults are commonly separated into two categories, "pneumonia" and "bronchitis," depending on whether the inflammation involves the alveolar spaces ("pneumonia") or the bronchi ("bronchitis"). In clinical practice, this precise distinction is rarely possible because many patients who clinically have only "bronchitis" may have x-ray evidence of alveolar involvement (consolidation or infiltrate). In practice, the less seriously ill patients, as described in this guideline, usually have primarily "bronchitis" and are managed as indicated. More seriously ill patients more often have "pneumonia" and require inpatient evaluation and management.

III. **Clinical features**

  A. **Symptoms**

   1. Cough is almost always present.

   2. The amount and character of sputum produced is of particular importance. Viral bronchitis rarely causes more than 2 tablespoons per day of sputum, which is mucopurulent. Bacterial bronchitis is frequently associated with purulent sputum, often more than 2 tablespoons per day.

   3. Chest pain, if present, is generally a substernal discomfort aggravated by coughing.

   4. There are no frank, shaking chills.

   5. Wheezing and slight dyspnea on exertion.

  B. Signs

   1. Temperature is usually less than 101°F. No tachypnea at rest.

   2. The chest is clear to percussion.

   3. Rhonchi or wheezing, or both, are present.

   4. Scattered rales may be present.

IV. **Laboratory and diagnostic studies**

  A. **Sputum**

   1. Sputum is initially clear in viral or mycoplasmal bronchitis, but purulent in bacterial bronchitis.

2. Gram stain and culture of sputum usually are not necessary unless sputum is purulent or pneumonia is suspected.

B. A chest x-ray may be taken if the clinical assessment is unclear, but generally is not necessary.

C. Blood count

1. A white blood cell count is indicated only if the clinical picture is unclear. Consult with physician.

2. The white blood cell count usually is normal in viral or mycoplasmal disease; the count is rarely elevated, even in bacterial infections.

V. Differential diagnosis

A. Pneumonia.

B. Tuberculosis and other chronic pulmonary diseases.

C. Bronchial asthma.

D. Congestive heart failure.

E. Uncommon causes of bronchitis such as Legionella, pertussis, etc.

VI. Treatment

A. Bronchitis with production of less than 2 tablespoons of mucoid or mucopurulent sputum per day.

1. Rest.

2. Aspirin or acetaminophen (Tylenol) for discomfort; see p. 159 for dosage.

3. Vaporizer or humidifier for moisture.

4. Cough suppressants, such as codeine or dextromethorphan hydrobromide, may be used sparingly.

   a. Codeine, 15–30 mg orally every 4–6 hours as needed (controlled substance—physician prescription required).

   b. Dextromethorphan hydrobromide, 30 mg orally every 6–8 hours as needed.

   and/or

5. Expectorants may be used, although there is debate as to their efficacy. Guaifenesin and terpin hydrate are available alone or in combination with cough suppressants:

   a. Guaifenesin, 200–400 mg every 4 hours as needed.

   b. Terpin hydrate, 200 mg every 4 hours as needed.

B. Bronchitis with production of more than 2 tablespoons of purulent sputum per day (usually associated with systemic symptoms).

1. Rest.

2. Aspirin or acetaminophen for discomfort (see p. 159 for dosage).

3. Expectorant (see **A.5**).

4. Vaporizer or humidifier for moisture; of most value in winter.

5. Antibiotic:

a. Erythromycin 250 mg orally qid × 10 days.

or

b. Ampicillin, 500 mg orally 4 times a day for 10 days.

or

c. Tetracycline, 250 mg orally 4 times a day for 10 days.

6. Bronchodilator (if significant wheezing is present)—aminophylline, 200 mg 4 times a day for 10–14 days.

7. Avoid bronchial irritants.

VII. Complications. Generally, none in simple bronchitis in adults.

VIII. Consultation-referral

A. Significant respiratory distress.

B. Failure to improve in 72 hours.

C. Elderly patients, particularly those with chronic cardiovascular or pulmonary diseases, who have evidence of worsening cardiovascular status. Patient should contact provider promptly for temperature greater than 102°F, increasing dyspnea or tachypnea, development of pleuritic pain, or if there is no improvement in 72 hours; or if patient is not well in 2 weeks.

Influenza: Adult

I. Definition. An acute contagious viral illness often occurring in epidemics and characterized by fever, malaise, myalgia, and respiratory symptoms.

II. Etiology. One or another of three myxoviruses having similar properties and categorized as influenza virus types A, B, and C. Influenza A viruses have shown an unusual ability to mutate, resulting in new antigenic strains that frequently produce worldwide epidemics.

III. Clinical features

A. Symptoms

1. Headache.

2. Malaise, lassitude, and occasionally prostration.

3. Myalgia.

4. Nonproductive cough.

B. Signs

1. Fever, often 102°–103°F.

2. Rhonchi and, occasionally, scattered rales.

IV. Laboratory studies. Generally, none.

V. Differential diagnosis

A. Other viral illnesses.

B. Bacterial pneumonia.

C. Other acute infectious illnesses.

VI. Treatment

A. Supportive therapy

1. Aspirin or acetaminophen, 325 mg, 2 tablets orally every 4–6 hours for fever and myalgia.

2. Increased fluid intake.

3. Mild cough suppressant, such as Robitussin-DM (guaifenesin and dextromethorphan hydrobromide), 2 teaspoons orally every 6–8 hours as needed.

B. Amantadine. In cases of influenza A, amantadine 100 mg orally BID for 4–7 days begun within 48 hours of onset of symptoms, is effective in shortening the duration of fever. Because there is no practical way to identify influenza A infection clinically, some practitioners empirically treat epidemic "influenza" with amantadine.

VII. Consultation-referral

A. Severely ill patients, particularly the elderly.

B. Respiratory distress or widespread rales or rhonchi on physical examination, or both of these.

C. Pregnant patients.

VIII. Follow-up. As needed.

Bronchial Asthma: Pediatric

I. **Definition.** A reversible obstructive airway disease characterized clinically by intermittent episodes of cough, dyspnea, and prolonged expiration with wheezing.

II. **Etiology.** Bronchial asthma may be of single, multiple, or unknown cause. The precipitating factor may not necessarily be the same in each episode. Each attack may be associated with one or a combination of the factors listed below:

A. Allergy—inhalant (dust, mold, pollen) or food (especially in infants).

B. Acute or chronic infection—viral, bacterial, fungal.

C. Weather changes—rising pressure and decreasing temperature, changes in humidity and wind velocity.

D. Extreme exertion.

E. Nonspecific irritants—chemical fumes, air pollution, tobacco smoke.

F. Psychogenic factors.

III. **Clinical features.** The amount of airway obstruction determines the severity of symptoms and signs.

A. **Symptoms**

1. Cough.

2. Dyspnea or chest tightness, anxiety, apprehension.

3. Wheezing.

4. Occasionally, vomiting following paroxysmal coughing.

5. Abdominal pain associated with coughing or respiratory distress.

6. Family history of allergic disease.

B. **Signs**

1. Prolonged expiration with expiratory and, occasionally, inspiratory wheezes.

2. Hyperresonant percussion note.

3. Tachypnea.

4. Sometimes, inspiratory and expiratory rhonchi or rales, or both.

5. Intercostal retractions.

6. Use of accessory muscles of respiration (e.g., sternomastoids and diaphragm).

7. Increased anteroposterior diameter of chest.

8. Cyanosis in severe attack.

9. Sometimes, with respiratory failure and decreased effort, less labored respirations, less audible wheezes.

10. Fever, if infection is present.

11. Evidence of upper respiratory tract infection.

12. Sometimes, evidence of other allergic diseases, such as allergic rhinitis and atopic dermatitis.

IV. Diagnostic studies. Chest x-ray only after consultation. X-ray is not needed in most cases.

V. Differential diagnosis

A. Acute bronchiolitis of infancy.

B. Aspirated foreign body (e.g., peanut), especially in young children with unilateral findings, although asthma can be associated with differences in findings in the two lung fields.

C. Bronchospasm associated with pneumonia.

D. Parasitic infestation (ascariasis, visceral larva migrans).

VI. Treatment

A. Moderate to severe acute attack

1. Administer aqueous epinephrine, 1:1000, for bronchodilatation:

   a. Inject 0.01 ml per kg (0.005 ml per lb), with a maximum dose of 0.3 ml, subcutaneously into the upper arm.

   b. If wheezes are still present after 20 minutes, repeat the dose of epinephrine. Do not delay the repeat dose beyond 20 minutes if no side effects are present. Delay the second dose if side effects (tremor, tachycardia, anxiety, sweating) develop.

   c. Document the effect of each dose by recording pulse, respirations, symptoms, auscultatory findings, and time of injection.

2. Try to calm and reassure the patient, because anxiety can increase bronchospasm.

3. Administer oxygen for cyanosis.

Table 6-1. Oral dosage of aminophylline (somophyllin) liquid (18 mg theophylline per ml)[a]

Body weight	Dose	Frequency
15–18 kg (33–40 lb)	4 ml	
18–22 kg (40–48 lb)	5 ml	
22–27 kg (48–59 lb)	6 ml	Every 6 hr. Continue for 2 weeks after all symptoms and signs have disappeared.
27–31 kg (59–68 lb)	7 ml	
31–35 kg (68–77 lb)	8 ml	
Over 35 kg (over 77 lb)	9 ml	

Note: Side effects include gastric irritation, nausea, vomiting, diarrhea, palpitations, headache, restlessness, and insomnia. Discontinue medication and consult physician should any of these occur.
[a]Tablets are less expensive than liquid. See Table 6-2 if child can swallow regular tablets or take chewable tablets.

4. Encourage increased oral fluid intake.

5. If the patient is not significantly relieved by the preceding regimen, consult the physician.

6. If the patient is significantly relieved and ready for discharge from the clinic, proceed with the following:

   a. Aqueous epinephrine suspension 1:200 (Sus-Phrine), for sustained (8–10 hours) bronchodilatation. Inject 0.005 ml per kg (0.0025 ml per lb) subcutaneously after shaking the vial; maximum dose is 0.15 ml.

   b. Maintenance therapy (see **B**).

B. Mild attack and home maintenance

1. Use theophylline preparation for bronchodilatation (see Table 6-1 or 6-2 for dosage).

2. Encourage intake of clear liquids.

3. Counsel patient to avoid precipitating factors that apply to that individual. Emotional stress and physical exertion should be avoided during an asthmatic attack, regardless of the underlying cause.

4. Suggest that the patient and family keep a record of when attacks occur to identify precipitating factors.

5. Oral antihistamines may be used in low dosages for relief of allergic symptoms (rhinitis, hay fever, etc.). There is no compelling evidence that they promote drying of respiratory secretions.

Table 6-2. Oral dosage of theophylline tablets

Body weight	Theophylline (Slo-Plyllin, 100 mg per tablet)	Aminophylline[a] (Aminophyllin, 100 mg per tablet)	Frequency
		Dose	
19–25 kg (42–55 lb)	1		Every 6 hr. Continue for 2 weeks after all symptoms and signs have disappeared.
25–31 kg (55–68 lb)		1½	
31–37 kg (68–81 lb)	1½		
37–45 kg (81–99 lb)		2	
Over 45 kg (over 99 lb)	2		

Note: Side effects include gastric irritation, nausea, vomiting, diarrhea, palpitations, headache, restlessness, and insomnia. Discontinue medication and consult physician should any of these occur.
[a]Aminophylline contains 85% theophylline.

VII. Complications of acute attack:

   A. Hypoxia.

   B. Atelectasis.

   C. Pneumonia.

   D. Dehydration.

   E. Pneumothorax or pneumomediastinum, or both.

   F. Respiratory failure.

   G. Death.

VIII. Consultation-referral

   A. Failure of acute attack to responds to treatment.

   B. Persistent wheezing at follow-up visit despite maintenance therapy.

   C. Side effects from theophylline therapy.

   D. Repeated attacks (more than two per year).

IX. Follow-up. Return visit in 10–14 days, or sooner if no improvement.

Bronchial Asthma: Acute Attack in a Known Adult Asthmatic

   I. Definition. A clinical syndrome characterized by episodes of wheezing cough and dyspnea due to reversible bronchospasm. Breathing in the intervals between acute attacks is virtually normal.

II. Etiology. An acute attack of bronchial asthma may be of a single, multiple, or unknown cause. Each attack may be associated with one or a combination of the factors listed below. The precipitating factor may not necessarily be the same in each episode.

A. Allergy—inhalant, food.

B. Acute or chronic infection—viral, bacterial, tuberculous, fungal.

C. Environmental physical factors—humidity, temperature, dust, fumes, odors.

D. Exertion.

E. Psychogenic factors.

III. Clinical features

A. Symptoms

1. History of frequent episodes of eczema or atopic dermatitis.

2. Cough.

3. Dyspnea.

4. Wheezing.

B. Signs

1. Prolonged expiration with expiratory and, occasionally, inspiratory wheezes.

2. Tachypnea.

3. Use of accessory muscles of respiration, such as sternomastoids and scalenus.

4. Intercostal retractions.

5. Perspiration.

6. Cyanosis, with severe asthma.

7. Hyperresonant percussion note.

8. Presence of the following, depending on etiology:

    a. Fever.

    b. Rhinorrhea.

    c. Evidence of upper respiratory tract infection or allergy.

IV. Laboratory and diagnostic studies

A. Pulmonary function studies. An objective measure of bronchospasm should be made in all cases.

1. Spirometry. Office spirometry can be used to establish the initial diagnosis of asthma, determine the severity of impair-

ment, evaluate the response to therapy, and evaluate the need for hospitalization. More commonly in office practice, the peak expiratory flow rate is used (see below).

2. Peak Expiratory Flow Rate (PEFR). Simple devices for measuring peak expiratory flow rate are available and can be used to quantitate the severity of the attack and measure responses to therapy. Criteria for severity in normal-sized adults are:

    a. 200 L/min. or greater—mild obstruction. Can usually be treated as outpatient.

    b. 100–200 L/min. Moderate obstruction. Usually should be held for observation of response to therapy in the office.

    c. 60–100 L/min. Severe obstruction. Hospitalization usually required.

B. If infection is suspected, the following should be initiated and a consultation obtained:

1. Chest x-ray, to demonstrate:

    a. Hyperinflation.

    b. Evidence of pulmonary infection.

    c. Cardiac enlargement and evidence of heart failure, if underlying heart disease is severe.

2. White blood cell count and differential count:

    a. Eosinophils may be elevated if allergic reaction is an important component of the asthma.

    b. If the white blood cell count is very high, acute infection should be suspected.

3. Microscopic examination of sputum:

    a. Gram stain of sputum showing polymorphonuclear leukocytes and bacteria should raise suspicion of acute infection.

    b. Wright's stain of sputum will show large numbers of eosinophils if allergic reaction is an important component of the asthma.

4. Culture of sputum:

    a. *Hemophilus influenzae* and pneumococcus are important pathogens.

    b. "Normal" flora (*Neisseria* and alpha-hemolytic streptococci) may be the cause of an acute attack.

V. Differential diagnosis

A. Acute bronchitis.

B. Aspirated foreign body.

C. Pneumonia.

D. Allergic reaction to drug, inhalant, or food (anaphylaxis), especially the syndrome of chronic sinusitis, nasal polyps, and asthma that is associated with aspirin ingestion.

E. Congestive heart failure (sometimes called *cardiac asthma*) may closely mimic allergic asthma.

F. Pulmonary emboli.

VI. Treatment. The following regimen is intended for young to middle-aged patients with known asthma and no heart disease.
Warning: Asthma may deteriorate into status asthmaticus in hours.

A. Ensure adequate hydration of patient by encouraging oral fluid intake.

B. Do not use sedatives without consulting physician.

C. Initially, inject 0.2–0.3 ml of 1:1000 aqueous epinephrine subcutaneously; reassess in 15–20 minutes and then repeat the dose if the attack persists. Up to 3 injections may be given, with assessment after each injection.

D. If epinephrine therapy **(C)** is successful:

   1. Inject 0.3 ml of aqueous suspension of epinephrine subcutaneously.

   2. Begin maintenance therapy:

   a. Aminophylline tablets, 200 mg every 6 hours or 4 times a day.

   or

   b. Theophylline tablets, 200 mg every 6 hours or 4 times a day.

   or

   c. Terbutaline sulfate tablets (Brethine), 5 mg every 8 hours or 3 times a day.

   Note: Recent evidence suggests considerable variation in the rates of absorption and metabolism of theophylline by patients who do not respond to usual suggested dosages. Rates can best be established by carefully monitoring blood levels of theophylline in these patients. Also, certain long-acting oral preparations may be used to advantage in some patients.

   3. Use antibiotics if infection is a significant component of the asthma:

   a. Erythromycin, 250 mg orally 4 times a day for 7 days.

or

    b. Ampicillin, 500 mg orally 4 times a day for 7 days (if patient is not allergic to penicillin).

  4. Expectorant, such as guaifenesin, is commonly used but of undocumented value.

  5. Continue inhalants, such as metaproterenol sulfate (Metaprel), if patient has been on them.

    Warning: Too-frequent use of inhalant therapy may worsen an asthmatic attack.

  6. Do not use cough suppressants and antihistamines without physician consultation.

E. If **A–D** are not successful, consult physician.

VII. Complications

A. Severe hypoxia.

B. Dehydration.

C. Atelectasis.

D. Pneumonia.

E. Pneumothorax or pneumomediastinum, or both.

F. Respiratory failure.

G. Side effects of bronchodilator drug therapy:

  1. Aminophylline or theophylline—related to excessive plasma levels (e.g., anorexia, nausea, vomiting, nervousness, headache, arrhythmia, convulsions).

  2. Terbutaline sulfate—tachycardia, nervousness, tremors.

VIII. Consultation-referral

A. All new cases, whether this is the patient's first attack or the first time the patient has been seen.

B. All asthmatics over 60 years of age.

C. All asthmatics with history of heart disease.

D. All patients known to have COPD, if any significant respiratory distress is present.

E. Peak expiratory flow rate < 100 L/min.

F. Patients in whom therapy fails.

G. Extreme shortness of breath.

H. Side effects of bronchodilator drug therapy (see **VII.G**).

IX. Follow-up. Patients should be followed regularly every 1–3 months and seen promptly whenever necessary for acute attacks or symptoms or signs of infection, or both.

Chronic Obstructive Pulmonary Disease (COPD): Adult

I. Definition. A complex syndrome of decreased pulmonary function made up of three components in various combinations: emphysema characterized by irreversible destruction of the distal airspace; bronchitis characterized by excessive mucus production and inflammation of the bronchi resulting in sputum production; and bronchoconstriction. Any of the three may predominate.

II. Etiology. Unknown. Most cases are strongly associated with a history of cigarette smoking. There are usually no symptoms for the first 10–20 years for the smokers who develop COPD. Mild dyspnea after exertion develops first and is followed by cough and sputum production. Serial testing of pulmonary function documents an increase over the expected loss of expiratory volume (FEV). Cessation of smoking does not restore the lost function but does decrease the rate of decline.

III. Clinical features

A. Symptoms

1. Significant impairment, as detected by spirometry, may be asymptomatic.

2. Shortness of breath, first noticeable with exertion.

3. Chronic cough and sputum production, frequently in the morning.

4. Often, episodes of wheezing.

B. Signs

1. Early, no signs on physical examination.

2. Tachypnea, somewhat labored, with loud breathing.

3. As the disease progresses, there are increasing signs of hyperinflation and obstruction, depending on the composition of the disease:

a. Increased anteroposterior diameter of the chest.

b. Hyperresonant percussion note.

c. Frequently, rhonchi.

d. Wheezing.

e. Distant heart sounds.

  f. Decreased lateral movement of the thorax, with increase in upward vector of the sternum.

  g. Decreased diaphragmatic movement.

  h. Use of the accessory muscles of respiration.

  i. Sometimes in severe disease, paradoxical inward movement of the lower costal margins.

 4. Signs of right-sided heart failure—peripheral edema, jugular venous distension, hepatomegaly.

IV. Diagnostic and laboratory studies

 A. Chest x-ray, only after physician consultation. Unsuspected pneumonia is common when there has been worsening of symptoms.

 B. Spirometry (FVC, FEV_1 and FEV_1/FVC).

 C. Sputum culture (occasionally helpful).

 D. Electrocardiogram.

 E. Arterial blood gas determination, after physician consultation.

V. Differential diagnosis

 A. Allergic asthma.

 B. Acute bronchitis.

 C. Congestive heart failure.

VI. Treatment

 A. Prevention. Complications in patients with known chronic obstructive pulmonary disease may be prevented by:

  1. Yearly immunization with influenza vaccine.

  2. Immunization with pneumococcal vaccine (Pneumovax) every 3 years.

  3. Cessation of smoking.

  4. Avoid any foods such as dairy products, spicy food, wine or other alcohol-containing beverages that in some people may increase bronchospasm and sputum.

  5. Avoid extremes in temperature.

  6. Home humidification of greater than 50% and 2–3 L of H_2O per day may help their secretions.

 B. Stable chronic disease

  1. Patient should **avoid pulmonary irritants,** especially cigarettes.

  2. Bronchodilator. Almost all patients with chronic obstructive pulmonary disease have some element of bronchospasm. Use an appropriate bronchodilator, such as

a. Aminophylline tablets, 200 mg every 6 hours or 4 times a day.

or

b. Theophylline tablets, 200 mg every 6 hours or 4 times a day.

or

c. Terbutaline sulfate tablets (Brethine), 5 mg every 8 hours or 3 times a day.

Note: Recent evidence suggests considerable variation in the rates of absorption and metabolism of theophylline by patients who do not respond to usual suggested dosages. Rates can best be established by carefully monitoring blood levels of theophylline in these patients. Also, certain long-acting oral preparations may be used to advantage in some patients.

d. Beta adrenergic agents by inhaler:

(1) Metaproterenol 1–3 puffs 94–6h.

(2) Albuterol 2 puffs 96h.

3. **Expectorants.** There is doubt as to whether these do more good than using a humidifier.

a. Glyceryl guaiacolate, 2 teaspoons by mouth every 4–6 hours.

b. Saturated solution of potassium iodide, 15 drops in a glass of water 3 times a day.

c. Vaporizer.

4. Patient should **avoid sedatives, antihistamines,** and **beta blockers.**

5. Patients with significant bronchitis should follow a routine of **postural drainage** 3 or 4 times a day.

a. Drink a hot cup of coffee or tea.

b. Use a vaporizer for 5–10 minutes.

c. Take an expectorant.

d. Proceed with postural drainage in four positions, staying in each position for 5 minutes:

(1) Supine.

(2) Right side down.

(3) Left side down.

(4) Prone, with head down at a 30-degree angle.

C. Acute attack of bronchitis (manifested by increased symptoms, fever, and change in color and quantity of sputum)

1. Consult physician.

2. General therapy as for chronic disease (see **B**).

3. Hydration and humidification (extremely important).

4. Antibiotics (if bacterial infection is suspected based on purulence of expectorated sputum).

a. Erythromycin, 250 mg orally 4 times a day for 10 days.

or

b. Ampicillin, 500 mg orally 4 times a day for 10 days (if patient is not allergic to penicillin).

c. Trimethoprim 160 mg/sulfamethoxazole 800 mg (Septra®, Bactrim®) one tablet orally twice a day for 14 days.

5. Chest x-ray, only after physician consultation.

VII. Complications

A. Pneumonia.

B. Respiratory failure.

C. Cor pulmonale.

D. Side effects of bronchodilator drug therapy; see Bronchial Asthma (Acute Attack in a Known Adult Asthmatic), **VII.G,** p. 176.

VIII. Consultation-referral

A. All new cases of suspected COPD.

B. Pneumonia.

C. Coexisting acute or chronic bronchitis, if the patient has any significant change in respiratory function or a temperature greater than 101°F.

D. Failure to improve within 48 hours.

E. Suspected respiratory failure, manifested by severe dyspnea or any confusion or clouding of consciousness, or both.

F. Side effects of bronchodilator drug therapy; see Bronchial Asthma (Acute Attack in a Known Adult Asthmatic), **VII.G,** p. 176.

IX. Follow-up

A. Acute attack. Telephone call if there is no improvement in 3 days, or immediately if condition worsens.

B. Stable chronic disease

1. In 3 months for review.

2. Repeat spirometry every year.

3. Development of symptoms or signs of respiratory infection or increased shortness of breath, or both. Emphasize to patient the importance of promptly consulting the nurse practitioner or physician.

Acute Bronchiolitis: Pediatric:

I. **Definition.** A generalized inflammation of the bronchioles, characterized by signs of expiratory obstruction, occurring usually as an epidemic disease in winter and early spring in children under 3 years of age.

II. **Etiology**

   A. Epidemic forms are usually caused by respiratory syncytial virus.

   B. Sporadic cases are usually viral in origin, but bacteria, allergy, and *Mycoplasma pneumoniae* may be responsible.

III. **Clinical features**

   A. Symptoms

     1. Onset as an upper respiratory tract infection.

     2. Paroxysmal coughing.

     3. Expiratory wheezing.

     4. Dyspnea.

     5. Difficulty sleeping and eating.

   B. Signs

     1. Rapid respirations.

     2. Symmetric expiratory wheezing or grunting, or both.

     3. Air-trapping causing liver to be pushed down, hyperresonant percussion note, and prolonged expiratory phase.

     4. Increased heart rate.

     5. Sometimes, fever (usually of low grade).

     6. Sometimes, rales.

IV. **Diagnostic studies.** Chest x-ray only after consultation. Usually, x-ray is not needed.

V. **Differential diagnosis**

   A. Pneumonia.

   B. Asthmatic bronchitis.

C. Tracheobronchitis.

D. Pertussis.

E. Aspirated foreign body, especially with unilateral signs.

VI. Treatment

A. Maintain adequate fluid intake.

B. Therapeutic trial of epinephrine after physician consultation when asthmatic bronchitis is suspected, as with recurrent episodes, older infant, or strong allergic family history.

C. Antibiotics are indicated only for complications such as acute otitis media.

VII. Complications

A. Hypoxia.

B. Progressive exhaustion followed by respiratory failure.

C. Dehydration from loss of water through lungs combined with poor intake (usually in infant under 4 months of age).

D. Superimposed bacterial infection, including acute otitis media associated with the accompanying upper respiratory disease.

VIII. Consultation-referral

A. Respiratory distress.

B. Children under 3 months of age.

C. More than two episodes. Refer to evaluation of possible underlying causes.

IX. Follow-up.

A. Phone contact in 24 hours.

B. Return visit if there is no improvement in 48 hours.

Pneumonia: Pediatric

I. **Definition.** Inflammation of the lung involving the alveoli or interstitial tissues, or both.

II. **Etiology**

A. A viral etiology is most common, particularly in preschool children. Respiratory syncytial virus and parainfluenza virus type 3 are particularly common causes in children under 3 years of age.

B. *Mycoplasma pneumoniae* probably accounts for at least half of the cases of pneumonia seen in school-age children, adolescents, and young adults. It is usually characterized by insidious onset and mild disease.

C. Bacterial pneumonia other than *Mycoplasma pneumoniae,* is less common than viral pneumonia and is usually due to pneumococcus, *Hemophilus influenzae,* or, rarely, *Staphylococcus aureus.* Marked toxicity and consolidation or pleural fluid are usually present.

D. *Chlamydia trachomatis* is a common cause of pneumonitis in the first 4 months of life.

III. Clinical features

A. Symptoms

1. Upper respiratory tract infection that precedes or accompanies the pneumonia.

2. Cough.

3. Fever.

4. Rapid or labored breathing, or both.

5. Lethargy.

6. Anorexia.

7. Abdominal pain and distention.

8. Vomiting.

B. Signs

1. Rapid breathing.

2. Labored breathing

    a. Grunting on expiration.

    b. Flaring of nostrils.

    c. Intercostal and subcostal retractions.

3. Fine, crackling rales.

4. Evidence of consolidation or pleural effusion, or both:

    a. Decreased breath sounds.

    b. Dullness to percussion.

5. Sometimes, marked fever, lethargy, and anorexia.

IV. Diagnostic studies. Chest x-ray only after consultation. X-ray is not needed in mild cases.

V. Differential diagnosis

A. Bronchiolitis and tracheobronchitis.

   B. Aspirated foreign body.

   C. Tuberculosis.

VI. Treatment

   A. Increased fluid intake.

   B. Rest, as needed.

   C. Acetaminophen (Tylenol) for fever (see Table 5-5, p. 151 for dosage).

   D. Antibiotics for bacterial, mycoplasmal, or chlamydial disease, after consultation.

   E. Avoid cough medications, particularly those which contain cough suppressants, in children.

VII. Complications

   A. Empyema.

   B. Atelectasis.

   C. Bronchiectasis.

   D. Pneumothorax.

   E. Dehydration.

VIII. Consultation-referral

   A. All cases of pneumonia.

   B. Failure to improve in 48 hours.

   C. Failure to resolve in 3 weeks.

IX. Follow-up

   A. Telephone call, home visit, or clinic visit every day until patient is afebrile and has no respiratory distress.

   B. Return visit in 3 weeks.

   C. Repeat chest x-ray for severe disease or persisting symptoms and signs. Consult physician for review of initial x-ray film for decision on the necessity for and timing of follow-up films.

Disorders of the
Cardiovascular System

Angina Pectoris: Adult

I. **Definition.** Pain, usually in the substernal region of the chest but occasionally in the epigastrium, neck, back, or arms, which is caused by an imbalance between the work required of the myocardium and the oxygen supply to the myocardium.

II. **Etiology.** Usually, atherosclerosis of the coronary arteries.

III. **Clinical features**

   A. **Symptoms.** Diagnosis is based primarily on the history of characteristic pain.

      1. **Location.** Pain is usually located in the substernal region of the chest, but occasionally is present in the epigastrium, neck, back, or arms.

      2. **Onset.** Pain occurs with an increase in the workload on the heart and is relieved by a decrease in the workload. Classically, this relation is demonstrated by pain occurring with work and relieved by rest (usually within 3–5 minutes).

      3. **Description.** The pain is usually described as squeezing or pressurelike, sometimes as expanding, and seldom as sticking, sharp, or burning.

      4. **Radiating pain.** Pain often radiates to the neck, shoulder, or arms (the left arm more often than the right).

      5. **Accompanying symptoms.** Sometimes there is slight shortness of breath, mild diaphoresis, or slight nausea, or a combination of these. The pain is not pleuritic.

   B. **Signs.** There may be no signs in uncomplicated angina. Nonetheless, one should carefully examine the heart and lungs for signs of congestive heart failure (CHF), valvular heart disease, etc.

IV. **Diagnostic studies.** ECG may show characteristic abnormalities, particularly during attack of pain. It may, however, be completely normal.

V. Differential diagnosis

   A. Acute myocardial infarction.

   B. Preinfarctional angina.

   C. Musculoskeletal pain (e.g., costochondritis).

   D. Esophagitis, esophageal spasm, and other gastrointestinal causes of chest pain.

   E. Pleurisy and other plumonary causes of chest pain.

   F. Psychosomatic chest pain.

   G. Malingering.

   H. Cervical spine root compression.

VI. Treatment. Angina pectoris can be divided into two broad categories, *stable angina* and *unstable angina,* which are treated differently:

   A. Stable angina is previously diagnosed angina that recurs with approximately the same amount of exertion with the same frequency and intensity of pain, and is relieved after approximately the same period of rest (less than 15 minutes).

   1. General measures:

   a. Reduction of the workload on the heart.

   (1) Reduction of exertion by the patient until attacks are infrequent or absent.

   (2) Reduction of workload by control of other diseases that tend to increase the workload.

   (a) Control of hypertension (see Uncomplicated Essential Hypertension [Adult], pp. 192–198).

   (b) Correction of anemia.

   (c) Treatment of anxiety.

   b. Improvement of cardiac performance without changing workload.

   (1) Treatment leading to compensation of CHF (see Congestive Heart Failure [Adult], **VI,** p. 189).

   (2) Correction of valvular heart disease.

   2. Specific therapy:

   a. Nitroglycerin, 1 tablet (0.3–0.4 mg) sublingually every 3–5 minutes until pain is relieved or headache results; not to exceed a total of 3 tablets.

      b. Long-acting nitrates. Consult physician.

      c. Beta blockers. Consult physician.

      d. Calcium channel blocking agents. Consult physician.

  B. Unstable angina consists of angina de novo (the first attack or attacks of angina) or a worsening of previously stable angina and is characterized by more severe or persistent pain, pain on less exertion, or pain at rest. These patients should be *referred* and hospitalization considered.

VII. Complications

  A. Myocardial infarction.

  B. CHF.

  C. Cardiac neurosis.

VIII. Consultation-referral

  A. Unstable angina, including angina de novo.

  B. Development of congestive heart failure.

  C. Elevated serum cholesterol and triglyceride levels.

  D. Angina requiring more than 3 nitroglycerin tablets for relief.

  E. Angina persisting more than 20 minutes.

IX. Follow-up and maintenance of stable angina

  A. Frequency of assessment. This frequency can vary considerably, depending on the severity of the disease and the presence of absence of other conditions, such as hypertension and CHF. For angina uncomplicated by other problems, a visit every 2–4 months should be adequate. *Any time angina becomes unstable (see* **VI.B**), *the patient should seek care.*

  B. Content of assessment

    1. Subjective evaluation:

      a. Stability of angina.

      b. Symptoms of CHF.

      c. Response to nitroglycerin, and complications such as headache.

    2. Objective evaluation:

      a. Assessment of heart and lungs, particularly for signs of CHF.

      b. ECG every two to three years.

Congestive Heart Failure (CHF): Adult

I. **Definition.** A complicated state of altered cardiac function in which there is inadequate cardiac output to meet the oxygen demand of metabolizing tissues, leading to excessive retention of salt and water.

II. **Etiology.** Any process that damages the heart. In the United States, the most common causes are arteriosclerotic heart disease and hypertensive heart disease.

III. **Clinical features**

   A. **Symptoms**

   1. Dyspnea on exertion.

   2. Orthopnea.

   3. Paroxysmal nocturnal dyspnea.

   4. Ankle swelling.

   5. Nocturia: In diabetes and congestive heart failure (CHF), patients pass large volumes of urine. In benign prostatic hypertrophy, there is frequent, difficult voiding of small amounts of urine.

   B. **Signs**

   1. Tachycardia.

   2. Weight gain, reflecting fluid retention.

   3. Neck vein distention.

   4. Rales, particularly over the base of the lungs.

   5. Gallop rhythm.

   6. Bilateral dependent edema.

   7. Hepatomegaly with severe, usually chronic, heart failure.

   8. Rarely, ascites.

IV. **Laboratory and diagnostic studies**

   A. Chest x-ray is indicated to confirm diagnosis and to better assess the magnitude of the problem.

   B. An ECG may be helpful in determining etiology; it is seldom helpful in establishing a diagnosis of failure or in monitoring response to therapy.

   C. Serum NA^+, K^+, HCO_3^-, Cl^-, and creatinine levels are useful as a baseline and should be measured before treatment is instituted.

D. Hematocrit or hemoglobin should be measured, because anemia may contribute to the pathogenesis of CHF.

V. Differential diagnosis

A. Other causes of dyspnea, such as chronic lung disease and asthma.

B. Other causes of edema, such as renal disease, liver disease, and local venous problems.

C. Recurrent pulmonary emboli.

D. Other causes of wheezing, such as asthma.

VI. Treatment. The general goal of therapy is to rid the body of excess salt and water by a combination of measures designed to **improve cardiac function** and to **increase renal excretion** of salt and water.

Note: Physician should be consulted before any treatment is begun.

A. Initial therapy

1. **Low-sodium diet.** Generally, few patients can restrict their sodium intake below 85 mEq per day without major alterations in their style of living and eating. Usually, however, restriction to this level is adequate. In refractory cases, further restriction should be attempted.

2. Measures to **improve myocardial function:**

   a. Reduction of systemic blood pressure to normal levels if it is elevated. Consult physician for regimen.

   b. Correction of anemia, if present.

   c. Use of digitalis preparations, such as digoxin. Consult physician for initial dosage regimen and establishment of maintenance therapy (see **IX.C.1**).

3. Measures to **increase renal excretion** of sodium and water:

   a. Oral diuretics if the patient is not acutely ill.

      (1) Hydrochlorothiazide, 25–50 mg every morning. The dosage may be increased to 100 mg every day.

      or

      (2) Chlorthalidone, 50–100 mg every morning.

      or

      (3) Furosemide, 20–40 mg every morning.

   b. Intramuscular diuretics (e.g., furosemide, 20–40 mg IM) should not be used without physician consultation.

B. Maintenance therapy (see **IX**).

VII. Complications

    A. Worsening CHF.

    B. Arrhythmias.

    C. Hepatomegaly, ascites, profound edema.

    D. Pulmonary embolism.

    E. Digitalis toxicity (see **IX.C.1**).

    F. Side effects of diuretics:

        1. Hypokalemia.

        2. Hyperglycemia.

        3. Hyperuricemia.

        4. Increased blood urea nitrogen (prerenal azotemia).

        5. Orthostatic hypotension.

    G. Pulmonary infection.

VIII. Consultation-referral

    A. All new patients should initially have a physician consultation.

    B. All patients should be followed by the nurse practitioner with close physician consultation until their condition is stable on a maintenance regimen. The nurse practitioner may then follow and alter the regimen as needed on the basis of the follow-up and maintenance guidelines (**IX**), but should consult frequently.

    C. Worsening CHF: In previously compensated patients who develop worsening CHF, consider these possible causes:

        1. Failure to adhere to low-sodium diet.

        2. Failure to comply with medical regimen.

        3. Progression or development of ischemic heart disease, even in the absence of pain.

        4. Failure to control blood pressure in hypertensive patients.

        5. Development of renal failure.

        6. Development of anemia.

    Appropriate evaluation of the etiology of worsening failure should be made prior to consultation with physician about management.

    D. Arrhythmia.

    E. Suspected digitalis toxicity.

IX. Follow-up and maintenance

    A. Frequency of assessment

1. Initial follow-up in 24 hours to determine if patient has improved.

2. Then every 1–2 weeks until patient is symptom-free and dry weight is achieved.

3. Then every month for 3 months.

4. Then every 6–8 weeks, indefinitely.

B. Content of assessment (related to basic diseases):

1. Subjective symptoms

   a. Dyspnea on exertion.

   b. Orthopnea.

   c. Paroxysmal nocturnal dyspnea.

2. Objective evaluation:

   a. Neck veins—look for distention.

   b. Chest examination—listen for rales.

   c. Cardiac examination—listen for gallop rhythm or arrhythmia.

   d. Abdomen—determine liver size.

   e. Extremities—check for edema.

   f. Weight (change in body weight is one of the most sensitive measurements of fluid balance).

3. **Laboratory tests**

   a. Blood urea nitrogen (BUN), serum creatinine, Na^+, K^+, HCO_3^-, and Cl^- initially; then BUN and K^+ at 2 weeks and 8 weeks; and then BUN and K^+ every 6 months if patient is stable.

   b. Hematocrit or hemoglobin, every year.

C. Treatment

1. **Digitalis** (Dosage or drug should not be altered without physician consultation.)

   a. Drug, most commonly used preparation, and maintenance dose is Digoxin, 0.125–0.375 mg orally every day.

   b. Assessment related to digitalis or digitalis toxicity.

   (1) Subjective symptoms (assess at each visit):

   (a) Nausea, vomiting, anorexia.

   (b) "Yellow vision," blurred vision.

        (c) Palpitations.

        (d) CNS symptoms (headache, disorientation, fatigue, malaise).

    (2) Objective signs (assess at each visit):

        (a) Bradycardia of 60 beats or less.

        (b) Arrhythmias, commonly premature ventricular contractions.

  2. Diuretics (dosage or drug should not be altered without physician consultation).

    a. Drugs and usual maintenance dosage:

      (1) Hydrochlorothiazide, 50–100 mg orally every day.

      or

      (2) Furosemide, 20–40 mg orally every day (occasional patient may require much larger dosage).

    b. Assessment related to possible side effects of diuretics:

      (1) Subjective symptoms (review at each visit):

        (a) Hypokalemia—lethargy, muscle cramps.

        (b) Gout—acute joint pain.

        (c) Diabetes—polyuria, polydipsia, weight loss.

      (2) Objective evaluation of orthostatic hypotension—obtain supine and standing blood pressure at each visit.

      (3) Laboratory tests:

        (a) BUN, serum creatinine, Na^+, K^+, HCO_3^-, Cl^- initially; then BUN and K^+ at 2 weeks and 8 weeks; and then BUN and K^+ every 6 months if patient is stable.

        (b) Uric acid, at 3 months and then annually.

        (c) Urinalysis for glucose; check if polyuria, polydipsia, or polyphagia develops.

Uncomplicated Essential Hypertension: Adult

  I. Definition. Persistent elevation of the arterial blood pressure greater than 150/100 mm Hg but less than 200/110 (present on weekly determinations over 1–3 weeks) without demonstrable cause and with no associated symptoms or signs of end-organ involvement.

  II. Etiology. Unknown.

III. Clinical Features

A. Symptoms

1. Usually, the patient is asymptomatic.

2. Hypertension of this magnitude can rarely be shown to be associated with the nonspecific symptoms that the general population associates with high blood pressure. The symptoms—dizziness, stuffiness, lightheadedness, and headaches—have not been found to be predictably present when blood pressure is elevated.

3. In uncomplicated hypertension, these symptoms of target organ involvement are not present:

   a. Symptoms of angina pectoris.

   b. Symptoms of congestive heart failure.

   c. Symptoms of cerebral ischemia or stroke syndrome.

   d. Severe headaches, nausea, and vomiting.

   e. Alterations in level of consciousness.

B. Signs

1. Elevation of arterial blood pressure greater than 150/100 mm Hg.

2. Sometimes, narrowing, copper-wiring, or arteriovenous nicking of the arterioles of the optic fundi. Usually there are no hemorrhages or exudates, and there is no papilledema.

3. Chest clear to percussion and auscultation.

4. The heart is usually normal, although it may show minimal to moderate left ventricular hypertrophy. No gallop rhythm is present.

5. No bruit over abdomen or flank or in back.

6. No edema.

7. Intact neurologic system.

8. No signs of Cushing's syndrome, hyperthyroidism, or pheochromocytoma.

IV. Laboratory and other studies

A. Before treatment

1. Blood urea nitrogen or serum creatinine.

2. Serium Na^+, K^+, HCO_3^- and Cl^- levels.

3. Blood sugar concentration (preferably 2 hours after eating, or after fasting).

    4. ECG.

    5. Chest x-ray.

    6. Urinalysis.

    7. Hypertensive intravenous pyelography, measurement of vanillylmandelic acid level, and other studies are deferred until the patient has been seen by the physician, or after consultation with the physician.

  B. After treatment. See **VI.C.**

V. Differential diagnosis

  A. Headaches and dizziness from other causes. Thought by patient to be a sign of hypertension.

  B. Secondary hypertension:

    1. Systolic hypertension:

      a. Arteriosclerotic vascular disease.

      b. Hyperthyroidism.

      c. Anxiety.

    2. Diastolic hypertension:

      a. Renal disease.

      b. Coarctation of aorta.

      c. Pheochromocytoma.

      d. Cushing's syndrome.

VI. Treatment. The goal of treatment is the achievement and maintenance of a reasonable blood pressure (less than 160/95) and the prevention of complications of either the disease or the treatment regimens.

  A. Step One therapy. If the patient meets the criteria as outlined for uncomplicated benign essential hypertension, proceed with the following:

    1. Salt-restricted diet. Salt intake should approximate 85 mEq (2 gm) sodium daily, but may be altered as necessary, depending on such factors as the patient's socioeconomic status, habits of living and eating, and ability to comprehend.

    2. Weight reduction.

    3. Thiazide diuretic.

      a. Hydrochlorothiazide:

        (1) Initial dosage is 50 mg orally every day.

(2) Dosage may be increased in 4–6 weeks to 50 mg orally twice a day or 100 mg orally every morning.

or

b. Chlorthalidone:

(1) Initial dosage is 50 mg orally every day.

(2) Dosage may be increased in 4–6 weeks to 100 mg orally every day.

Note: Thiazide diuretics cause renal potassium loss. If a patient is on digitalis, supplemental potassium should be given after renal function is established. If patient is not on digitalis and serum potassium stays above 3.0 mEq per liter, potassium need not be given. Because many patients do not need supplemental potassium and are maintained on only one drug, we do not advocate using a formulation that combines Thiazide with triamterene, a weak diuretic that decreases potassium loss. These combination drugs are expensive and necessitate two drugs where one is usually sufficient.

B. Step Two therapy. If Step One therapy is not effective in bringing the blood pressure to normal levels, one should begin Step Two therapy while maintaining the previously established dose of thiazide diuretic (Step One therapy).

A wide variety of drugs are available for Step Two therapy. For nurse practitioner practice, we still recommend that reserpine be the drug of first choice (see orders below) because it is effective, inexpensive, produces few side effects, and is safe. It should always be given with the thiazide diuretic. Several thiazide-reserpine combination tablets are available and can be recommended because administration of a single once-a-day tablet often improves compliance.

Our second choice for Step Two therapy is a beta blocking agent. We do *not* feel these agents should be initially prescribed by the nurse practitioner without M.D. consultation due to the number of side effects and complications of therapy. Once maintenance dosage is established, however, we feel nurse practitioners can safely monitor patients. (See order below for side effects of beta blockers.) Other antihypertensives are frequently used at this level and many physicians may prefer another drug. In fact it is likely that Step Two therapy will be dramatically changed in the near future.

1. Reserpine—Begin with reserpine 0.125 mg p.o. q.d. May increase to 0.25 mg p.o. q.d. in one if needed. Higher doses are not recommended.

C. Follow-up and maintenance—general

1. Frequency of assessment

a. Every 1-2 weeks until normal blood pressure is achieved.

b. Then every month for 3 months.

c. Then every 6 months, indefinitely.

2. Content of assessment (related to hypertension)

a. Subjective symptoms:

(1) Headaches.

(2) Dizziness.

(3) Angina.

(4) Congestive heart failure.

(5) Cerebral ischemia or stroke syndrome.

(6) Nausea, vomiting.

(7) Alterations of level of consciousness.

b. Objective evaluation:

(1) Blood pressure—measure supine and standing at each visit.

(2) Appropriate examination related to symptoms.

(3) Routine examination of heart, lungs, and nervous system every 6 months.

3. Assessment related to thiazide

a. Subjective symptoms (review at each visit):

(1) Hypokalemia—lethargy, muscle cramps.

(2) Gout—acute joint pain.

(3) Diabetes—polyuria, polydipsia, weight loss.

b. Objective evaluation:

(1) Orthostatic hypotension—obtain supine and standing blood pressure at each visit.

(2) Serum potassium level—measure initially; repeat after diuretic dose is established; and repeat every 6 months thereafter.

(3) Serum uric acid level—check any time joint pain develops. Check at end of the first 3 months of therapy, and then annually.

(4) Blood sugar level—check routinely at end of the first 3 months of therapy and then annually, 2 hours after eating. Check if polydipsia, polyuria, or polyphagia develops.

4. Assessment related to reserpine

   a. Subjective symptoms:

   (1) Nasal stuffiness.

   (2) Depression.

   (3) Epigastric pain.

   (4) Impotence.

   b. Objective evaluation—obtain a stool for occult blood and hematocrit prior to consultation if patient has epigastric pain or symptoms such as melena suggesting gastrointestinal bleeding.

5. Assessment related to maintenance of patients on beta blockers

   a. Subjective symptoms:

   (1) Tiredness.

   (2) Fatigue.

   (3) Depression.

   (4) Nausea.

   (5) Shortness of breath.

   b. Objective symptoms:

   (1) Pulse rate should be taken to ensure that beta blockage has occurred. Patients who remain hypertensive but who have a resting pulse above 80 may not be taking their medicines or may require a higher dose.

   (2) If significant side effects are noticed, physician should be consulted about the appropriate course of action. Do *not* abruptly discontinue beta blockers, because rebound hypertension or angina or both can occur.

VII. Complications

   A. Angina pectoris.

   B. Congestive heart failure.

   C. Transient cerebral ischemia or other stroke syndrome.

   D. Secondary renal disease.

    E. Complications of therapy.

VIII. Consultation-referral

    A. Any patient with hypertension who has a sustained blood pressure of 170/110 mm Hg while on therapy, or any patient exhibiting signs of complications of hypertension.

    B. Any patient not controlled on maximum dosage of thiazide or re-serpine plus a thiazide.

    C. Any patient who has complications related to the treatment reg-imen.

IX. Follow-up. See **(VI.C)**.

Chronic Occlusive Arterial Disease of the Extremities: Adult

  I. Definition. A disease characterized by a chronic decrease in blood flow to one or more of the extremities due to partial or complete occlusion of one or more of the peripheral blood vessels.

  II. Etiology. Usually, atherosclerosis. Congenital lesions, trauma, and other mechanisms may be causative. The condition frequently is associated with diabetes.

 III. Clinical features

    A. Symptoms. Symptoms, depending on the site of occlusion, in the buttocks, thigh, calf, or arm:

      1. Intermittent claudication (cramping pain in the muscles on exercise that is relieved by rest).

      2. Occasionally, nocturnal muscle cramps.

      3. Feeling of coldness in involved extremity.

    B. Signs

      1. The involved extremity may demonstrate any or all of these:

        a. Decreased pulses.

        b. Coolness.

        c. Loss of hair.

        d. Shiny, atrophic skin.

      2. Ischemic necrosis (gangrene) in advance disease.

      3. Bruits may be heard over the involved vessel, particularly the femoral arteries and abdominal aorta.

 IV. Laboratory studies

   A. Appropriate urine sugar or blood sugar determination, or both, to screen for diabetes mellitus.

   B. Fasting serum cholesterol and triglyceride levels.

V. Differential diagnosis

   A. Raynaud's disease.

   B. Raynaud's phenomenon.

   C. Scleroderma.

   D. Problems of venous stasis; see Stasis Ulcer of the Lower Extremity (Adult), p. 200.

VI. Treatment

   A. The patient should be instructed in methods of good skin care using lanolin, lamb's wool between toes, and properly fitting shoes.

   B. The patient should be cautioned about the dangers of excessive heat or cold.

   C. Vasodilating drugs are of no proven benefit and need not be prescribed. Consult with physician for patients who are on medications previously prescribed by another physician.

   D. The patient should avoid cigarette smoking and ingestion of caffeine.

VII. Complications

   A. Gangrene, ulceration.

   B. Impaired nail and hair growth.

VIII. Consultation-referral

   A. All patients should be discussed with the physician or referred within 2 weeks for evaluation regarding further diagnostic studies and consideration for revascularization.

   B. Any patient with acute onset of symptoms should be referred that day.

   C. Patients with gangrene or skin ulcers should be referred.

IX. Follow-up

   A. All patients should be seen every 3-6 months to follow their circulatory status; physician should be consulted if there is progression of the disease.

   B. All patients should be instructed to return if symptoms increase or if skin abrasions, lacerations or other breaks in skin surface, inflammation, or infection occur.

Stasis Ulcer of the Lower Extremity: Adult

   I. **Definition.** A chronic ulcerative lesion of the lower extremity caused by poor circulation due to venous stasis.

  II. **Etiology.** Chronic impairment of venous return secondary to varicose veins, a previous episode of thrombophlebitis, or congestive heart failure.

 III. **Clinical features**

   A. **Symptoms**

   1. Pain at the ulcer site.

   2. History of varicose veins or thrombophlebitis.

   3. History of congestive heart failure.

   B. **Signs**

   1. A chronic ulcer of the lower extremity with minimal surrounding inflammation or infection.

   2. Associated varicose veins.

   3. Usually, pitting edema of the involved leg.

   4. Frequently, brawny edema.

   5. Negative Homans' sign.

   6. Intact peripheral pulses in the involved extremity.

  IV. **Laboratory studies.** None.

   V. **Differential diagnosis**

   A. Chronic lymphedema.

   B. Arterial occlusive lesion (see Chronic Occlusive Arterial Disease of the Extremities [Adult]).

  VI. **Treatment**

   A. Rest and elevation of the involved leg.

   B. Muscular activity of elevated leg by such measures as using a footboard during bed rest.

   C. Initial vigorous cleansing of the ulcer by the nurse practitioner followed by twice-daily cleansing of the ulcer by the patient at home, using povidone-iodine (Betadine) and water, or hydrogen peroxide. Apple dry dressing after cleansing. A povidone-iodine soak may be necessary before beginning cleansing.

   D. Application of Unna's paste boot if measures **A–C** do not result in healing in 3 weeks, particularly if the patient is unable or unwilling to follow the regimen.

VII. Complications

    A. Severe extension of ulcer.

    B. Cellulitis.

VIII. Consultation-referral

    A. Surrounding inflammation or infection.

    B. Positive Homans' sign.

    C. Failure to heal within 1 month.

  IX. Follow-up. Return visit every 5–7 days until ulcer is healed or consultation is required.

Disorders of the Gastrointestinal System

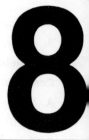

Aerophagia (Gaseous Distention Syndrome): Adult

I. **Definition.** A syndrome characterized by gaseous distention of the abdomen, which is usually worse after meals and relieved in part by eructation or passage of flatus.

II. **Etiology.** Most of the offending gas is due to air-swallowing. Most of these patients suffer from tension-anxiety states.

III. **Clinical features**

 A. **Symptoms**

 1. Abdominal distention.

 2. Mild, nonlocalized abdominal discomfort.

 3. Eructation and passage of flatus, often with partial relief.

 4. Often, worsening of symptoms just after meals.

 5. No nausea or vomiting.

 6. No change in bowel habits.

 B. **Signs**

 1. No weight loss.

 2. No fever.

 3. Minimal, nonlocalized abdominal tenderness.

 4. Slight to moderate abdominal distention with hyperresonance to percussion.

 5. No fluid wave or shifting dullness.

 6. No masses or visceromegaly.

 7. Normal to slightly hyperactive bowel sounds.

 8. Negative rectal examination.

IV. **Laboratory studies**

A. Negative stool guaiac test.

B. Normal hematocrit.

V. Differential diagnosis

A. Intestinal obstruction.

B. Ascites.

C. Mesenteric vascular insufficiency.

VI. Treatment

A. Reassurance and explanation of the nature of the problem.

B. Simethicone (Mylicon), 40–50 mg, 1 or 2 tablets chewed with each meal.

VII. Complications. None.

VIII. Consultation-referral. Symptoms persisting more than 4–6 weeks.

IX. Follow-up. Return visit if there is no improvement.

Constipation: Pediatric

I. Definition. Difficulty in passing stools, commonly associated with excessive firmness of stools and a decrease in frequency of defecation.

II. Etiology

A. Acute constipation (a change of a few days' to several months' duration from a pattern that was within normal limits)

1. Pain on defecation with secondary retention of stools:

a. Anal fissure.

b. Anal irritation from diaper dermatitis.

c. Rarely, perianal abscess.

2. Functional causes

a. Acute illnesses, especially if associated with decreased appetite and activity (e.g., upper respiratory tract infection in an infant).

b. Uncomfortable circumstances for defecation (e.g., outdoor toilet in cold weather, unfamiliar location of toilet facilities, school where permission is required).

c. Emotional upset.

d. Disruption of usual daily routine.

3. Hard stools

    a. Drying of stools retained because of the conditions cited in 1 and 2.

    b. Recent change to a constipating diet (e.g., excessive milk products or chocolate and not enough fruits or vegetables or other foods with significant residue).

B. Chronic constipation

  1. Psychogenic stool-holding.

  2. Chronic neuromuscular disease.

  3. Aganglionic megacolon (Hirschsprung's disease).

III. Clinical features. Depending on the underlying cause, any of these features may be present:

A. Symptoms

1. Acute constipation

    a. Pain on defecation if stool is hard, or anal fissure or irritation is present, or both.

    b. Straining on defecation.

    c. Firm stools.

    d. History of blood-tinged stool if anal fissue is present.

    e. Decrease in frequency of defecation from usual pattern.

    f. No vomiting.

    g. Mild abdominal pain, if any.

2. Chronic constipation

    a. Psychogenic stool-holding:

      (1) Onset in infancy or early childhood.

      (2) Huge bowel movements at long intervals.

      (3) Encopresis.

      (4) Evidence of behavior problems.

    b. Aganglionic megacolon:

      (1) Occasionally, onset is in newborn period.

      (2) Rare spontaneous passage of formed stool.

      (3) No encopresis; however, "overflow" diarrhea may occur.

      (4) Anorexia and vomiting in early infancy.

B. Signs

1. Acute constipation

    a. Physical examination is usually normal.

    b. Anal fissure, marked diaper dermatitis, or perianal abscess may be present.

    c. Mild abdominal distention with palpable firm stool is apparent on abdominal and rectal examination.

  2. Chronic constipation

    a. Psychogenic stool-holding:

      (1) Rectum is large and filled with soft stool.

      (2) Mild abdominal distention may be present.

      (3) Remainder of physical examination usually is normal.

    b. Aganglionic megacolon:

      (1) Rectum usually is empty.

      (2) Abdominal distention with palpable stool masses may be present.

      (3) Growth may be poor.

IV. Laboratory studies. None.

V. Differential diagnosis

  A. Normal patient. Parents may not appreciate or accept the wide variation of patterns of defecation that are within normal limits.

  B. Intestinal obstruction. Abdominal pain and vomiting usually are present.

VI. Treatment

  A. Acute constipation

    1. Treat underlying cause:

    a. Diaper dermatitis (see Chapter 3, Diaper Dermatitis).

    b. Anal fissure:

      (1) Warm sitz baths.

      (2) Gentle cleansing with soap and water.

      (3) Petrolatum to anus.

      (4) Nonconstipating diet in older children (see **2**).

    c. Reassure parent if constipation is associated with an acute self-limiting illness.

    d. Encourage parents to help child avoid or cope with environmental or emotional circumstances that promoted constipation.

2. **Prescribe a nonconstipating diet:**

   a. Add 2 tablespoons of dark corn syrup to 1 quart of infant's milk formula.

   b. Decrease milk intake of older child to less than 1 pint a day

   c. Increase intake of fresh vegetables, fruit juices, and fruits especially prunes, raisins, figs, and dates (apples and ba nanas are least helpful).

3. **Remove fecal impaction,** if present:

   a. Manual removal.

   b. Pediatric Fleet enema.

B. **Chronic constipation.** Consult with physician.

VII. **Complications**

A. **Acute constipation**

1. Fecal impaction.

2. Overresponse of parents, whose excessive, abnormal concern with and manipulation of child's bowel function can lead to be havior problems, encopresis, stool-holding, and parent-child in teraction problems.

B. **Chronic constipation**

1. Fecal impaction.

2. Secondary behavior and psychosocial problems.

3. Failure to thrive and colitis (due to aganglionic megacolon).

VIII. **Consultation-referral**

A. Chronic constipation.

B. Recurrent fecal impaction.

C. Failure to respond to treatment.

Constipation: Adult

I. **Definition.** Properly defined as excessive *hardness* of stool without regard to frequency of bowel movements. Normal frequency of bowel movements can vary greatly, from two or three movements daily to one every 3–5 days; however, a decrease in frequency from the pa tient's usual routine may be significant.

II. **Etiology**

A. Opiates.

B. Barium following x-ray contrast studies.

C. Dehydration.

D. Debilitation in chronically ill persons.

E. Bed rest.

F. Colonic cancer.

G. Hypothyroidism.

III. Clinical features

A. Symptoms

1. Increased hardness of stool or difficulty in moving bowels.

2. Decreased frequency of bowel movement; this is not important if stools are soft and not difficult to pass, unless the decrease in frequency has been a recent change.

3. Sometimes, abdominal distention.

4. *No abdominal pain* in simple constipation.

5. No nausea or vomiting.

6. No history of blood in stools.

B. Signs

1. *No abdominal tenderness* on palpation.

2. Normal bowel sounds (absence of bowel sounds does *not* occur in simple constipation).

3. No hyperactive rushes or tinkles.

4. Fecal impaction may ocur, particularly in bedridden, debilitated, or elderly patients.

5. Sometimes, palpable fecal material. Feces feel firm, but may be indented. No other intra-abdominal mass may be molded.

IV. Laboratory and other studies

A. Stool specimen, if obtained, is negative for occult blood.

B. X-ray or other studies are not indicated for simple constipation.

V. Differential diagnosis

A. Failure of bowels to move because of intestinal obstruction or ileus.

B. Hypothyroidism.

C. Neurotic preoccupation with bowel function (rather than true constipation).

VI. Treatment

A. Check for the presence of fecal impaction in elderly or debilitated patients. (Remember that fecal impaction often presents as diarrhea.)

B. Patient should increase water intake.

C. Patient should drink warm water or coffee early in the morning to initiate bowel movement.

D. Patient should increase intake of fruits, bulky vegetables, or cereals.

E. If measures **A–D** do not work, the patient can try the following medications (starting with the milder agents, listed first):

   1. Psyllium hydrophilic mucilloid (Metamucil), 1–2 teaspoons in glass of water 2 or 3 times a day.

   2. Milk of magnesia, 15–30 ml before bed with sufficient fluids (contraindicated in patients with chronic renal disease).

   3. Dioctyl sodium sulfosuccinate (Colace), 100 mg twice a day.

F. Rarely, an enema is necessary for relief of severe constipation in chronically ill patients.

   1. Saline solution, 1–2 liters rectally.

   2. Soapsuds, 1–2 liters rectally.

   3. Adult Fleet enema.

VII. Complications

A. Hemorrhoids.

B. Rectal fissures.

C. Fecal impaction.

VIII. Consultation-referral

A. Any suspicion of an acute abdominal condition.

B. Abdominal pain or tenderness.

C. Nausea or vomiting associated with failure to move bowels.

D. Hyperactive bowel sounds, or rushes or tinkles.

E. Absence of bowel sounds.

F. Occult blood in stool.

G. Failure to respond to conservative treatment (as outlined in **VI**).

IX. Follow-up.
Patients should be followed until "normal" bowel function resumes, that is, passage of soft stool without difficulty, because failure to improve may indicate more serious underlying illness.

Simple Diarrhea: Adult

I. Definition. Frequent loose or watery stools that are not bloody, purulent, or greasy in character.

II. Etiology

  A. Infections (usually, acute viral infections).

  B. Psychophysiologic disturbances (often related to stress).

  C. Dietary indiscretion.

  D. Laxatives.

III. Clinical features

  A. Symptoms

   1. Frequent loose or watery stools.

   2. Sometimes, mild crampy abdominal pain just prior to bowel movement.

   3. Absence of gross blood.

   4. Epidemiology: Knowledge of similar cases occurring in the community is very helpful in making a diagnosis of viral gastroenteritis.

  B. Signs

   1. Low-grade or no fever.

   2. Abdomen may show slight diffuse tenderness. No localized tenderness. No rebound or referred rebound tenderness.

   3. Hyperactive bowel sounds.

   4. No high-pitched rushes or tinkles.

IV. Laboratory and other studies

  A. Stool guaiac test is negative.

  B. Methylene blue stain of fecal specimen for white blood cells. Presence of significant numbers of white blood cells suggests bacterial etiology.

  C. Studies such as barium enema should be done only after consultation.

  D. Stool culture or testing of stool for ova and parasites initially is not necessary.

V. Differential diagnosis

  A. Bloody diarrhea

    1. Certain infections.

    2. Regional enteritis.

    3. Ulcerative colitis.

    4. Diverticulitis.

    5. Certain bowel cancers.

  B. Steatorrhea. Malabsorption syndrome.

VI. Treatment

A. Symptomatic management

    1. Kaolin and pectin (Kaopectate), 60–90 ml after each loose bowel movement.

     or

    2. Paregoric, 1 teaspoon orally every 4 hours, not to exceed 6 teaspoons in 24 hours.

     or

    3. Diphenoxylate HCl and atropine sulfate (Lomotil), 1 or 2 tablets 4 times a day until diarrhea stops, not to exceed 8 tablets in 24 hours.

     or

    4. Loperimide (Imodium) 4 mg (2 capsules) orally followed by 2 mg (one capsule) orally after each loose stool not to exceed 16 mg (eight capsules) in 24 hours.

B. Clear liquid diet of tea, carbonated beverages, or soups until improvement.

VII. Complications

  A. With simple diarrhea—generally, none.

  B. With severe diarrhea—dehydration, vascular collapse, or shock.

VIII. Consultation-referral

  A. Bloody stools.

  B. Positive methylene blue stain for fecal leukocytes.

  C. Abdominal tenderness or rebound tenderness.

  D. High fever or toxicity.

  E. Dehydration.

  F. Weight loss greater than 5% of body weight.

  G. Recurrent or chronic diarrhea (diarrhea persisting 5–7 days).

IX. Follow-up. Return visit if no improvement within 48 hours.

Functional Bowel Disease (Irritable Colon Syndrome): Adult

I. **Definition.** A syndrome characterized by frequent passage (up to 4–6 movements per day) of small amounts of loose, watery stool associated with mild lower abdominal discomfort and a frequent sensation of a need for further defecation recurring in tense, anxious patients, particularly at times of stress.

II. **Etiology.** In some manner, tension and anxiety in susceptible patients produce increased intestinal motility and decreased transit time, leading to frequent loose, watery stool. The bowel itself is not inflamed and appears normal on examination. The disturbance is in bowel function.

III. **Clinical features**

   A. **Symptoms**

      1. Frequent passage (up to 4–6 movements per day) of loose, watery stool.

      2. Mild lower abdominal discomfort, often preceding and relieved by defecation.

      3. No nausea or vomiting.

      4. No history of blood in stools.

      5. Stools often contain mucus.

   B. **Signs**

      1. No weight loss.

      2. No fever.

      3. Minimal lower abdominal tenderness.

      4. No rebound or referred rebound tenderness.

      5. Normal to slightly hyperactive bowel sounds.

      6. No masses or visceromegaly.

IV. **Laboratory studies**

   A. Stool guaiac test is negative.

   B. Hematocrit reading is normal.

   C. Stool examination for ova and parasites is negative.

V. **Differential diagnosis**

   A. Inflammatory bowel diseases (e.g., ulcerative colitis and regional enteritis).

   B. Infectious causes of diarrhea.

   C. Parasitic infestations.

   D. Tumors of the large bowel.

VI. Treatment

   A. Reassurance as to the nature of the problem.

   B. Reduction of stress in life situation.

   C. Mild tranquilizer, after physician consultation.

   D. Antidiarrheal agents, such as paregoric or Lomotil, are not indicated.

VII. Complications. None.

VIII. Consultation-referral. Failure to improve in 4–6 weeks.

   IX. Follow-up. Return visit if no improvement in 3–4 days.

Acute Gastroenteritis: Pediatric

   I. Definition. An acute inflammation of the gastrointestinal tract characterized by passage of stools that are more liquid than normal, usually with an increase from the patient's normal frequency. The disorder is often preceded by or associated with vomiting.

  II. Etiology

   A. Often of unknown cause. Many cases are due to rotavirus infection.

   B. Occasionally due to the following:

   1. Specific **bacterial infection.**

   a. *Shigella* (relatively common in some areas).

   b. *Salmonella.*

   c. *Campylobacter.*

   d. *Yersinia.*

   2. Side effect of **oral antibiotics.**

   3. Food poisoning.

   a. *Salmonella.*

   b. Staphylococcal enterotoxin (not an actual infection).

   4. Parasitic infestation.

   a. *Giardia lamblia.*

  III. Clinical features

   A. Symptoms

1. Increased liquid content of stools with no specific color change.

2. Increased frequency of stools.

3. Vomiting.

4. Abdominal pain.

5. Sometimes, coexisting respiratory tract infection or otitis media.

6. Sometimes, flecks of blood in stool as diarrhea continues.

7. With dehydration—listlessness and lethargy.

8. Sometimes, family history of similar illness.

B. Signs

1. Sometimes, low-grade fever.

2. Abdominal distention (usually mild).

3. Abdominal tenderness (usually generalized, but may be more prominent in any area).

4. Increased bowel sounds.

5. With dehydration—sunken eyes, dry mucous membranes, decreased skin turgor, and weight loss.

IV. Laboratory studies

A. Usually, none are necessary.

B. Stool culture for bacteria should be done if any of these apply:

1. Blood-tinged mucus in stool.

2. Fever over 102°F rectally or 101°F orally.

3. Family or closed population outbreak.

4. Diarrhea persisting over several days.

V. Differential diagnosis

A. **Normal patient.** Parents may not appreciate or accept the wide variation of patterns of defecation that are within normal limits.

B. **Intussusception.** This usually occurs in a patient aged 3–24 months who has a sudden onset of severe, paroxysmal abdominal pain and vomiting. It may be followed within 8–12 hours by loose stools containing blood and mucus.

C. **Appendicitis.** Rarely, a pelvic appendix can cause diarrhea if appendicitis develops.

VI. Treatment

A. **General management.**

1. Explain to parents that there is no specific therapy to stop symptoms immediately but that attention to diet and fluid management (see **3**) is needed. Discourage use of antidiarrheal and antiemetic medications.

2. Search for early signs of dehydration:

   a. Instruct parents to record nature and amount of fluid intake, occurrence of vomiting, the number and character of stools, and frequency of urination.

   b. Weigh the patient carefully at the initial visit and each follow-up visit to determine the state of fluid balance. Infants should be weighed naked, and older children, with the same, minimal clothing at each visit.

   c. Examine for sunken eyes, dry mucous membranes, and decreased skin turgor.

3. Dietary management of mild diarrhea and vomiting may be varied, depending on age (older children are less likely to progress to dehydration) and rapidity of improvement. Advise parent on these guidelines:

   a. First 12 hours

   (1) Discontinue present diet, including milk.

   (2) Drinking small amounts of clear liquids with low electrolyte concentration, such as cola or ginger ale (at room temperature without carbonation) may decrease the tendency to vomit. Offer every 2–4 hours.

   b. Next 12 hours. Increase amounts of clear liquids.

   c. Next 24 hours

   (1) If diarrhea has *not* improved, continue with clear liquids. In children under 3 years of age, alternate feedings of an electrolyte solution (Pedialyte or Lytren) with the clear liquids. If improvement then results, proceed to step **(2)**.

   (2) If diarrhea has improved, add easily absorbed solids (e.g., Jell-O, salt crackers, or bananas) to the clear liquid diet.

   d. If diarrhea continues to improve after 48 hours of clear liquids and the simple solid foods listed in **(2)**, the following foods may be gradually added: dry toast, baked potato (without butter), infant cereal mixed with water instead of milk, and more Jell-O.

   e. Milk, cheese, eggs, and fried foods should be withheld until it is certain the foods in **d** are tolerated well.

   f. If milk exacerbates the diarrhea; consult the physician if the patient is a young infant (for whom milk is the major food in the diet).

B. Bacterial gastroenteritis:

    1. Proceed with treatment outlined in **A.**

    2. Consult with physician about the need for antimicrobial therapy (e.g., antibiotic therapy for *Shigella*).

C. Side effects of oral antibiotics:

    1. Diarrhea is usually mild, and the antibiotic may be continued unless diarrhea increases.

    2. If diarrhea increases:

        a. Consult physician about substituting an alternative antibiotic and consideration of enterocolitis due to clostridium difficile toxin or staphylococcus aureus.

D. Food poisoning.

    1. Proceed with treatment outlined in **A.**

    2. Consult physician about the need for further management, including epidemiologic investigation.

VII. Complications. Complications, which are more likely to occur in infants than in older children, include:

    A. Dehydration.

    B. Hypovolemic shock.

    C. Inability to tolerate milk during recovery period (probably due to secondary lactase deficiency).

VIII. Consultation-referral

    A. Vomiting and diarrhea in children under 3 years of age.

    B. Dehydration.

    C. Severe abdominal pain.

    D. Moderate amount of blood in stools (more than just flecks).

    E. Failure to improve with treatment within 48 hours.

    F. Inability of a young infant to tolerate return of milk formula to diet.

    G. Bacterial infections or food poisoning.

    H. Chronic diarrhea.

IX. Follow-up

    A. Under 3 years of age. Return visit or telephone call daily until patient improves.

    B. Over 3 years of age. Return visit in 48 hours or sooner if there is no improvement.

Hiatal Hernia with Esophagitis: Adult

  I. Definition. Herniation of the stomach through the diaphragm. Hiatal hernia is generally asymptomatic unless associated with esophagitis due to reflux of acid into the esophagus.

  II. Etiology. Unknown.

 III. Clinical features

    A. Symptoms

      1. Burning substernal pain that is worse when bending over or lying down, particularly after meals. Pain often relieved by antacids.

      2. May experience regurgitation of acid into posterior pharynx, particularly when lying down.

    B. Signs. Physical examination is usually normal, but patient may have minimal tenderness on palpation of the epigastrium.

 IV. Laboratory studies

    A. Hematocrit or hemoglobin is normal.

    B. Stool guaiac test is negative.

  V. Differential diagnosis

    A. Strictures (secondary to lye ingestion, carcinoma, stomach tubes).

    B. Pains of myocardial infarction or other nongastrointestinal problems.

    C. Peptic ulcer.

    D. Esophagitis of other causes.

 VI. Treatment. Advise patient to:

    A. Eat frequently.

    B. Avoid food 2 hours before bedtime.

    C. Take antacids, 2 tablespoons (30 cc; 1 oz) 1 hour after meals and just before bedtime,

      or

      Alginic acid antacid tabs (Gaviscon®)—two to four tablets chewed and swallowed 1 h. p.c. and hs.

    D. Elevate head of bed on 6- to 8-inch blocks.

    E. Reduce weight.

F. Avoid tight clothing around the abdomen and chest.

G. Anticholinergics, theophylline, beta adrenergic agents, diazepam, meperidine, nicotine, and calcium channel blocking agents all may exacerbate reflux and should be avoided.

VII. Complications

A. Gastrointestinal bleeding.

B. Anemia.

C. Aspiration.

D. Structure formation.

VIII. Consultation-referral

A. Gastrointestinal bleeding.

B. Persistent symptoms.

C. Severe anemia.

D. Weight loss.

E. Dysphagia.

F. Vomiting.

IX. Follow-up

A. Weekly, until patient is asymptomatic; then whenever necessary for recurrence of symptoms.

B. Barium swallow and upper gastrointestinal x-ray series, if symptoms change (after consultation with physician).

Uncomplicated Duodenal Peptic Ulcer Disease: Adult

I. Definition. Ulceration of duodenal mucosa producing pain but *not* bleeding or obstruction.

II. Etiology. The etiology is unknown, but peptic ulceration can be related to the following factors:

A. Neuropsychiatric disorders

1. Stress.

2. Personality trait.

B. Endocrine disorders. These conditions are related to increased hydrochloric acid production:

1. Hyperparathyroidism.

2. Zollinger-Ellison syndrome.

C. Drugs

1. Aspirin.

2. Nonsteroidal anti-inflammatory agents such as indomethacin, phenylbutazone, ibuprofen, piroxicam, naproxen, sulindac, tolmetin, meclofenamate.

3. Reserpine

4. Corticosteroids such as prednisone.

D. Other diseases

1. Cirrhosis.

2. Pancreatitis.

3. Pulmonary disease.

4. Arthritis.

III. Clinical features

A. Symptoms

1. Abdominal pain (in epigastrium or right upper quadrant), usually 1–2 hours after meals (sooner, if gastric ulcer is present).

2. Pain relief with food and antacids.

3. Occurrence of pain at night but not just before breakfast.

4. Intermittent nausea, vomiting, and belching.

5. No history of hematemesis or melena.

B. Signs

1. Direct epigastric tenderness without rebound or referred rebound tenderness.

2. Normal stool with *no* melena on rectal examination.

IV. Laboratory and other studies

A. Hematocrit.

B. Negative test for occult blood in stool.

C. Upper gastrointestinal x-ray series for atypical pain patterns and in males over 45 years with onset of new symptoms (after consultation with physician).

V. Differential diagnosis

A. Funcational disease.

B. Hiatal hernia.

C. Coronary insufficiency.

D. Gastric ulcer.

   E. Less frequently, mild pancreatitis and biliary colic.

VI. Treatment. Advise patient on these measures:

   A. Diet. Small, frequent feedings. Fats, milk, and cream are not necessary and only increase the risk of atherosclerosis. Avoid caffeine, strong spices, alcohol, and cigarettes.

   B. Antacids. 2 tablespoons (30 cc; 1 oz) 1 hour and 3 hours after meals and at bedtime.

   C. Cimetadine (Tagamet) or ranitidine (Zantac). Use only after consultation with physician.

   D. Sucralfate (Carafate). Use only after consultation with physician.

   E. Anticholinergics. Rarely used; consult physician.

VII. Complications

   A. Gastrointestinal bleeding.

   B. Perforation of the stomach or duodenum and development of peritonitis.

   C. Intractable pain.

   D. Obstruction.

VIII. Consultation-referral

   A. Failure of antacids to relieve symptoms in 2 weeks.

   B. Gastrointestinal bleeding manifested by melena, occult blood in stool, or a drop of more than 4% in the hematocrit reading, even in the absence of recognized bleeding.

   C. Progressive weight loss.

   D. Signs and symptoms of an acute abdominal condition, including rigidity and rebound or referred rebound tenderness.

   E. All gastric ulcers.

IX. Follow-up

   A. Every 2 weeks for 4 weeks after acute onset of symptoms of pain (without gastrointestinal bleeding) to check for:

   1. Response of pain to antacids.

   2. Evidence of gastrointestinal bleeding (history of hematemesis or melena or positive test for occult blood in stool.

   B. Check for side effects of antacids, such as diarrhea and constipation. Watch for development of congestive heart failure in elderly patients if Maalox, Gelusil, or other antacids with high sodium content are used (Riopan has a low sodium content).

C. An upper gastrointestinal series generally is not necessary in the clinical follow-up of duodenal ulcer that becomes asymptomatic.

D. After 6–8 weeks of effective antacid therapy (relief of symptoms), antacids may be stopped and regular usage resumed only if symptoms recur.

Hemorrhoids (Piles): Adult

I. **Definition.** Varices of the hemorrhoidal veins, which drain the area of the anus, are called hemorrhoids. Internal hemorrhoidal veins and internal hemorrhoids occur on the mucosal side of the mucocutaneous junction; external hemorrhoidal veins and external hemorrhoids occur on the skin side.

II. **Etiology.** The principal cause of hemorrhoids is loss of support of the connective tissue of the anus and dilation of the submucous veins, resulting in the formation of varicosities of the hemorrhoidal veins. Often, such factors as position, straining at stool, and occupation are thought to contribute to the pathogenesis of hemorrhoids.

III. **Clinical features**

A. Acute external hemorrhoids

1. **Symptoms.** Constant mild pain, itching, and irritation aggravated by defecation and sitting.

2. **Signs**

   a. Bluish, firm (thrombosed) varix protruding around the anus and covered with skin. May occupy only a small portion of area around anus or may surround it entirely.

   b. Bleeding occurs from an external hemorrhoid if the varix ruptures.

B. Chronic external hemorrhoids.
May appear as painless swellings around anus, which appear when patient strains at stool, then disappear. The stretching of skin over repeated acute episodes of thrombosis may leave a redundancy of tissue, or an "appendage," after the acute state has resolved. These "appendages" are easily seen and palpated and are called tags.

C. Acute internal hemorrhoids

1. **Symptoms**

   a. If not prolapsed through anus, bleeding may be only symptom. Bleeding from internal hemorrhoids is bright red blood, usually occurring at the end of defecation. The blood may actually drip into the toilet bowl.

b. With prolapse and thrombosis, patient may have severe pain.

2. Signs

   a. Normally, not visible externally.

   b. Through an anoscope, appear as soft, red-to-purple varices just proximal to the mucocutaneous junction.

   c. When prolapse occurs, hemorrhoids protrude through anus and resemble an external thrombosed varix.

   Note: A patient with hemorrhoids usually has a combination of both external and internal types. Internal hemorrhoids are responsible for painless bleeding; either can cause painful swelling.

D. Chronic internal hemorrhoids

   1. Symptoms

   a. Painless bleeding; see **III.C.1.**

   b. Occasional prolapse occurs with straining or long standing and is easily reduced. Generally, there is little pain.

   2. Signs. Most often there is no external evidence of internal hemorrhoids in chronic painless state (see **III.C.2.**).

IV. Differential Diagnosis

   A. Prolapse of internal hemorrhoids must be differentiated from thrombosis of external hemorrhoids (internal hemorrhoids should be pushed through anus).

   B. Condyloma acuminatum (venereal wart).

   C. Condyloma latum (a lesion of secondary lues).

V. Laboratory. Generally, none, unless severe bleeding occurs; then a hematocrit is indicated.

VI. Treatment

   A. Chronic external hemorrhoids. No treatment is necessary.

   B. Acute thrombosed hemorrhoids

   1. Early. Surgical consultation.

   2. After 24–48 hours. Conservative treatment (advise patient on the following measures):

   a. Stay off feet; prone position is preferred as much as possible.

   b. Sitz bath for 20 minutes 3 times a day.

      c. Liquid diet.

      d. Stool softener, such as Colace or Metamucil.

C. Chronic internal hemorrhoids

  1. Protrusion. Reinsert into rectum.

  2. Bleeding. Decrease straining at stool by using stool softener, such as Colace, 100 mg twice daily. If diarrhea is present, use antidiarrheal agent (see Simple Diarrhea [Adult] **VI.A,** p. 210).

  3. May use **rectal suppositories,** such as Preparation H or Anusol, which are astringents.

D. Acute thrombosis of internal hemorrhoid with prolapse requires physician consultation.

VII. Complications

  A. Bleeding and subsequent anemia.

  B. Necrosis or thrombosis with ulceration.

VIII. Consultation-referral

  A. Acute thrombosed internal hemorrhoid if severe, of if there is prolapse of internal hemorrhoid.

  B. Chronic bleeding that has caused anemia.

  C. Conservative treatment is ineffective.

IX. Follow-up. As needed for recurrence of symptoms.

Disorders of the Genitourinary System

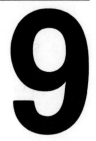

Cystitis: Adult Female

I. Definition. A condition characterized by inflammation of the bladder, marked by dysuria and frequency, and not accompanied by systemic complaints. It is frequently seen in females at the onset of sexual activity. Dysuria and frequency, without fever or flank pain, may be associated with a number of problems (see **Differential**). Previously a culture of 100,000 colonies per high-powered field was thought necessary to prove bacterial infection; however, counts as low as 1,000 colonies per high-powered field of pathogenic bacteria occur, with urinary tract infection limited to bladder and urethra.

II. Etiology

A. Bacteria are identified in 60–70% of patients with symptoms of cystitis; of these, *Escherichia coli* is the most frequently encountered in the ambulatory population. *Staphylococcus saprophyticus*, a gram's positive organism, has been identified in a small number of patients. The bacteria originate in the gastrointestinal tract. Women with recurrent urinary tract infection may have increased adherence of pathogenic bacteria to vaginal vestibule prior to infection. Entrance to the bladder is through the urethra; sexual activity may milk bacteria into the bladder.

B. Occasionally nonbacterial pathogens such as *Chlamydia* are identified.

III. Clinical features

A. Symptoms

1. Dysuria, frequency, urgency.

2. Occasionally, gross hematuria.

3. Occasionally, low back or lower abdominal pain. No flank or costovertebral pain.

4. No shaking chills.

5. Usually, no gastrointestinal complaints.

  6. No vaginal or urethral discharge.

B. Signs

  1. No fever, or temperature less than 100°F.

  2. Only slight lower abdominal tenderness.

  3. No peritoneal signs.

  4. Normal bowel sounds.

  5. No costovertebral angle tenderness.

IV. Laboratory studies. Urine for examination must be collected carefully (see Urinary Tract Infection [Pediatric], **IV.A.1**, p. 230). A clean-catch urine specimen is particularly important for females because of the possibility of vaginal contamination. If epithelial cells appear in a clean-catch urine specimen, the specimen has been contaminated.

  A. Urinalysis. White and red blood cells and bacteria may be present.

   1. Greater than 10 white blood cells per high-power field has only a 50% correlation with cultures of 100,000 colony-forming units, but has a much better correlation with lower counts (10^{2-4}) of colony-forming units.

   2. The presence of any bacteria in an unspun urine specimen has a high correlation with significant cultures.

  B. Urine culture. A colony count >1000 of a single urinary tract pathogen per milliliter may indicate an infection. If bacteria or significant WBC's or both are present and symptoms clearly indicate cystitis that is not a relapse (see **V.A.1**), then cultures need not be done. If there is a problem of relapse or a complicated history, cultures should be obtained.

V. Differential diagnosis

  A. Recurrent attack of cystitis. Patient may symptomatically appear to have cystitis, but if attacks are recurrent an effort should be made to differentiate between relapse and reinfection.

   1. Relapse

    a. Usually occurs within a few weeks after previous infection.

    b. Bacteria obtained from culture are the same as that from the previous episode.

    c. Bacteria obtained from urine may be antibody coated, which indicates kidney involvement.

    d. Suggests pyelonephritis, anatomic abnormality, or nephrolithiasis that provides a focus for infection that has been inadequately treated.

   e. May require a long course of antibiotics.

 2. Reinfection

   a. Occurs sporadically, with no relation to previous infection.

   b. Bacteria obtained from urine are not the same as that found during previous infection.

   c. Bacteria are not antibody coated.

   d. Suggests infection limited to bladder from reentry of bacteria from below.

   e. Responds rapidly to a wide variety of antibiotics. Recent studies suggest that a single dose of amoxicillin may be sufficient.

B. Acute pyelonephritis. Patient is sick. Although dysuria and frequency are present, these symptoms are overshadowed by systemic complaints of high fever and flank pain. Patient has occasional shaking chills. Occasionally pyelonephritis may cause only lower-tract complaints.

C. Vaginitis. Complaints are predominantly vaginal, with accompanying dysuria and frequency.

D. Urethritis. Dysuria is the chief complaint; a discharge, which may be purulent, is present (an unusual finding in females).

E. Acute abdominal disorder. Severe abdominal pain and rebound tenderness, which are not found in cystitis, are present.

F. Cervicitis

G. Salpingitis

VI. Treatment

A. Relapse should be referred to physician.

B. Initial occurrence or obvious reinfection:

 1. Recent studies indicate that a single dose of either sulfisoxazole, sulfamethoxazole and trimethoprim (Septra, Bactrim), or amoxicillin is effective in treating cystitis. This maneuver also may separate patients with lower-tract infection from those with upper-tract disease; those which recur after single-dose therapy may have upper-tract disease and need to be more closely evaluated. Use single-dose treatment if:

   a. Symptoms less than 3 days.

   b. Vaginitis or overt upper-tract infection is not present.

   c. No complicating factors exist such as diabetes, urinary-tract stones, anatomic abnormalities, pregnancy, or recurrent infection.

        d. Patient can be relied upon for follow-up visits.

    2. Antibiotics. Treatment may be instituted with any of these:

        a. Amoxicillin, 3.0 grams orally in one dose.

        b. Four tablets, each containing trimethoprim 80 mg and sulfamethoxazole 400 mg (Bactrim, Septra).

        For patients with symptoms of cystitis for whom single-dose therapy is not indicated, one of these may be used:

        c. Sulfisoxazole (Gantrisin), 1 gm orally 4 times a day for 10 days. This is the drug of choice in previously untreated cystitis.

          or

        d. If patient is allergic to sulfonamides, use trimethoprim, 100 mg twice a day for 10 days.

C. Urinary infections in pregnancy

    1. Cystitis. Treatment is the same as outlined in **C** and **D**, but the following precautions should be taken during pregnancy:

        a. Ampicillin may be used at all stages of pregnancy.

        b. Cephalexin (Keflex), 250 mg 4 times a day for 10 days, may be used in patients who are allergic to ampicillin.

        c. Nitrofurantoin macrocrystals (Macrodantin), 100 mg 4 times a day for 10 days, may be used in patients allergic to ampicillin, but not after 36 weeks in gestation or if any renal impairment is expected.

        d. Sulfisoxazole (Gantrisin) may be used up to 30 weeks in gestation.

        e. Septra (or Bactrim) and tetracycline should not be used.

    2. Pyelonephritis of pregnancy. Patients with symptoms of pyelonephritis require immediate consultation and often need hospitalization for parenteral antibiotics.

VII. Complications

    A. Chronic infection.

    B. Pyelonephritis.

VIII. Consultation-referral

    A. Failure to improve in 3 or 4 days.

    B. Recurrent cystitis:

        1. Reinfection within 2 weeks.

   2. More than three episodes in one year.

   C. Growth of original pathogen on follow-up urine culture.

   D. All males with cystitis.

   E. Patient with diabetes or known kidney stones.

IX. **Follow-up.** Urine cultures are expensive. If patient is asymptomatic, urine cultures need not be obtained routinely after antibiotic therapy has been completed.

Acute Pyelonephritis: Adult

   I. **Definition.** An infectious disease involving the collecting system and the renal parenchyma of the kidney.

   II. **Etiology.** Bacterial infection, usually with a gram-negative organism; *Escherichia coli* is the most common.

III. **Clinical features**

   A. Symptoms

      1. Dysuria, frequency, urgency. (These are primarily symptoms of cystitis, but they may be present in pyelonephritis.)

      2. Usually, flank pain.

      3. Often, frank, shaking chills.

      4. Often, nausea or vomiting, or both.

      5. No vaginal or urethral discharge.

   B. Signs

      1. Usually, fever of 101°F or higher.

      2. Tenderness on percussion over costovertebral angle.

      3. Negative abdominal examination except for tenderness to deep palpation in the involved flank area.

      4. Patient generally has systemic illness and appears very sick.

   IV. **Laboratory studies** (use clean-catch urine specimens).

      A. Urinalysis shows white blood cells (frequently in clumps), white cell casts, proteinuria, and red blood cells.

      B. Urine culture shows a colony count greater than 100,000 of the urinary tract pathogen.

   V. **Differential diagnosis**

      A. Cystitis.

      B. Prostatitis.

C. Other causes of flank or back pain. (The general public commonly and erroneously considers back pain as tantamount to kidney infection.)

VI. **Treatment.** These measures are for an initial occurrence of acute pyelonephritis in an otherwise healthy patient; all patients require at least a consultation and any complicated patient requires a referral. If patient is feeling well enough to care for himself or herself, can take oral medicines, and is not dehydrated, therapy can be instituted at home. Hospitalization may be required for systemically ill or septic patients or those with complicating diseases such as diabetes.

   A. **Antibiotics** (ask the patient whether he or she is allergic to the drug):

   1. Ampicillin, 500 mg orally 4 times a day for 10 days.

   B. The patient must be followed closely. If vomiting becomes a problem, intramuscular medications are necessary.

   C. Antibiotics may need to be changed on the basis of clinical response and results of sensitivity testing of the organism.

VII. **Complications.** Chronic pyelonephritis.

VIII. **Consultation-referral**

   A. Severely ill or toxic patient; patient requiring intramuscular medications.

   B. Diabetic patient.

   C. Elderly or debilitated patient.

   D. Any recurrence.

   E. Positive culture obtained in follow-up (see **IX.B** and **C**).

IX. **Follow-up**

   A. The patient should be in telephone contact in 24 hours and then every day until asymptomatic.

   B. A repeat urine culture is carried out 1 week after cessation of treatment.

   C. A second repeat culture in about 6 months is desirable.

Urinary Tract Infection: Pediatric

I. **Definition.** A bacterial infection of the kidneys, collecting system of the kidneys, or bladder, or a combination of these. It includes significant asymptomatic bacteriuria.

II. Etiology

A. Approximately 80% of cases are due to *Escherichia coli.*

B. The remainder are usually due to *Klebsiella, Proteus mirabilis, Enterobacter, Staphylococcus epidermidis,* enterococci, or *Pseudomonas.*

III. Clinical features

A. Epidemiology

1. Newborn infants. Significant bacteriuria is more common in males than females and has an overall frequency of about 1%.

2. Preschool children. Symptomatic urinary tract infection is relatively common in this age group. Urinary tract infection in general is 10–20 times more common in females than males.

3. School-age children. Symptomatic urinary tract infection is less frequent than in the preschool period, but at least one episode of significant asymptomatic bacteriuria will occur in at least 5–6% of females between 6 and 17 years of age. The prevalence of asymptomatic bacteriuria is 30 times greater in females. Asymptomatic bacteriuria is associated with increased risk of symptomatic infection in the future.

B. Symptoms

1. The infection may be completely asymptomatic and discovered on routine screening for bacteriuria.

2. Urinary tract symptoms may be present:

a. Urgency, frequency, dysuria.

b. Enuresis in a child who had achieved control.

c. Flank pain.

d. Suprapubic pain.

e. Foul-smelling or cloudy urine.

f. Occasionally, hematuria in acute cystitis.

3. Various combinations of other symptoms, with or without urinary tract symptoms, may be present:

a. Gastrointestinal symptoms, such as anorexia, nausea, and vomiting.

b. Abdominal pain.

c. Lethargy, irritability.

d. Unexplained fever.

C. Signs

1. Often, normal physical examination; asymptomatic bacteriuria is discovered on routine screening.

2. Suprapubic tenderness.

3. Costovertebral angle percussion tenderness.

4. Fever, alone or with other signs and symptoms.

5. Failure to thrive.

IV. **Laboratory studies.** *The diagnosis of a urinary tract infection is based on the finding of significant growth of bacteria from a urine culture.*

A. **Urine culture**

1. **Collection of specimen** (written instructions* should be available for parents, or trained personnel should assist in collecting specimen).

   a. Urine specimen should be collected in a sterile container after the urethral meatus and surrounding area have been thoroughly sponged with an ordinary liquid soap solution and rinsed with water-soaked sponges. Four soaped sponges followed by four rinse sponges should be used for females and wiping direction should be from front to back. One soaped sponge and one rinse sponge are sufficient for males after the foreskin of uncircumcised males is retracted.

   b. After infancy, a clean-voided *midstream* urine specimen should be collected.

   c. Specimen should be cultured immediately after it is collected. If there is any delay, store specimen in refrigerator.

   d. Drug sensitivity studies for potential urinary pathogens should be requested.

2. **Minimal diagnostic criteria**

   a. Two consecutive clean-voided specimens revealing 100,000 or more of the same, single urinary pathogen per milliliter of urine are diagnostic.

   b. If only one specimen for culture can be obtained before symptoms require therapy, urinalysis should reveal abundant bacteria in order to make a preliminary diagnosis of urinary tract infection.

   c. Lower colony counts (10,000–100,000 organisms per milliliter) *may* represent infection, especially in patients with recurrent or chronic urinary infections, in patients on sup-

---

*For details see Calvin M. Kunin, *Detection, Prevention and Management of Urinary Tract Infections* (2nd ed.). Philadelphia: Lea & Febiger, 1974, pp. 53–72.

pressive but inadequate antibiotic therapy, and in patients who are emptying their bladders frequently. When the count is between 10,000 and 100,000 organisms per milliliter, culture should be repeated.

    d. A colony count of fewer than 10,000 organisms per milliliter usually indicates contamination.

    e. Cultures producing colony counts of 100,000 or more per milliliter of mixed organisms should be repeated, as they suggest contamination in a patient who has not had urinary tract instrumentation.

B. Urinalysis on a clean-voided specimen (examine urine as soon as possible):

    1. More than 20 bacteria per high-power field in the sediment of a centrifuged specimen usually indicate the presence of 100,000 or more organisms per milliliter.

    2. Pyuria *alone* is *not* a reliable guide to the presence of an infection:

        a. Pus cells may be contaminants from the vagina and vulva.

        b. Pyuria is absent in up to 50% of patients with significant bacteriuria.

        c. Pyuria may persist for several days after an infection has been successfully treated.

        d. There are other diseases that cause sterile pyuria.

    3. Urine should be examined for other elements—cast, red blood, cells, protein, sugar, specific gravity, pH.

V. Differential diagnosis

A. Vulvovaginitis.

B. Urethritis.

C. Prostatitis (in postpubertal male).

D. Nonbacterial cystitis (e.g., hemorrhage cystitis associated with adenovirus type 11).

VI. Treatment. Consultation is required *before* instituting treatment for a urinary tract infection (see **VIII**). Treatment, after consultation, will usually consist of:

A. Antibiotic. Usually, an oral sulfonamide is prescribed (see Table 9-1 for dosage of sulfisoxazole (Gantrisin) suspension. Be certain the patient is not allergic to the drug.

B. Ample fluid intake and frequent voiding.

VII. Complications

Table 9-1. Oral dosage of sulfisoxazole (Gantrisin) suspension (500 mg per 5 ml)

Body weight	Initial dose given in clinic	Subsequent doses	Frequency
5–7 kg (11–15 lb)	500 mg (5 ml)	250 mg (2.5 ml)	
7–9 kg (15–20 lb)	600 mg (6 ml)	300 mg (3 ml)	
9–12 kg (20–26 lb)	800 mg (8 ml)	400 mg (4 ml)	
12–15 kg (26–33 lb)	1000 mg (10 ml)	500 mg (5 ml)	
15–18 kg (33–40 lb)	1200 mg (12 ml)	600 mg (6 ml)	4 times a day for 10 days
18–22 kg (40–48 lb)	1500 mg (15 ml)	750 mg (7.5 ml)	
22–25 kg (48–55 lb)	1800 mg (18 ml)	900 mg (9 ml)	
Over 25 kg[a] (over 55 lb)	2000 mg (20 ml)	1000 mg (10 ml)	

[a]Patients weighing over 25 kg (55 lb) who are able to swallow tablets safely may be given sulfisoxazole (Gantrisin) tablets (500 mg per tablet), 1000 mg (2 tablets) 4 times a day for 10 days.

    A. Failure to control infection because organism is resistant to antibiotic prescribed.

    B. Marked systemic toxicity (high fever, vomiting), with possible bacteremia associated with pyelonephritis. Patient may not be able to tolerate oral therapy.

    C. Recurrent infection. In school-age girls, 80% of patients will have at least one recurrence of significant bacteriuria, which may or may not be symptomatic.

    D. Rarely, chronic infection, with progressive renal damage. Patients at risk are usually discovered when radiologic study of the urinary tract is performed.

VIII. Consultation-referral. A consultation is required before instituting treatment for a urinary tract infection.

    A. If patient is asymptomatic or only mildly symptomatic, consultation may be requested after the results of the urine cultures are known.

    B. If patient is moderately or markedly symptomatic, consultation should be requested after the results of urinalysis are known.

    C. A consultation is again required at the follow-up visit 2 or 3 days after treatment has been started under the following circumstances:

1. Patient is still symptomatic.

2. Original urine cultures were not diagnostic of urinary tract infection.

3. Antibiotic sensitivity studies reveal resistance to prescribed drug.

IX. **Follow-up**

A. After 2 or 3 days of therapy:

1. Assessment of clinical status.

2. Review original culture results.

B. If medication is changed at the first follow-up visit, a return visit is again needed in 2 or 3 days for clinical assessment.

C. One week after completing a course of antibiotic therapy:

1. Assessment of clinical status.

2. Urinalysis on clean-voided specimen.

3. Urine culture and antibiotic sensitivity testing.

D. *If no further infections occur,* the following schedule of visits for clinical assessment, urinalysis, and urine culture is required:

1. After one month.

2. Then every 6 months for one year.

3. Then routine health maintenance visits.

E. Consultation should be requested 6–8 weeks after treatment has been completed for an intravenous pyelogram and a voiding cystourethrogram.

Primary Gonococcal Infections: Adult

I. **Definition.** Gonococcal infection of the genitourinary tract, oropharynx, or anorectum. Urethral infections may be accompanied by asymptomatic pharyngeal or rectal infection in those who have orogenital contact. Occasionally pharyngitis or proctitis may be the presenting complaint.

II. **Etiology.** *Neisseria gonorrhoeae.*

III. **Clinical features**

A. **Males.** Primary infection may be urethral, pharyngeal, or anorectal.

    1. Occasionally, asymptomatic.

    2. Urethritis (most frequent acute presentation) begins acutely only a few days after exposure.

        a. Dysuria and frequency.

        b. Purulent discharge.

    3. Pharyngitis from orogenital contact.

    4. Anorectal infection:

        a. Anorectal burning.

        b. Mucopurulent discharge.

        c. Painful bowel movements.

B. Females. Primary infection may be urethral, endocervical, pharyngeal, or anorectal.

    1. Occasionally, asymptomatic.

    2. Urethritis (dysuria, frequency).

    3. Salpingitis:

        a. Bilateral lower abdominal pain.

        b. Adnexal tenderness.

        c. Tenderness with manipulation of cervix.

        d. Elevated temperature and chills in some cases.

        e. Occasionally, females with gonococcal infections will develop pain in the right upper quadrant.

    4. Pharyngitis from orogenital contact.

    5. Anorectal infection (see **A.4**).

IV. Laboratory studies

    A. Gram stain of urethral discharge in both male and female.

    B. VDRL test for syphilis.

    C. Culture in cases unproved by gram stain. Culture area under suspicion—pharynx, anus, urethra, endocervix. (For urethral culture, insert small swab or wire several centimeters into meatus.) Endocervix is best site for screening in females. In patients with urethritis and history of orogenital exposure, consider culture of pharynx and rectum to detect asymptomatic disease. Gonococcal infections in these areas have a high failure rate to amoxicillin, ampicillin, or spectinomycin.

V. Differential diagnosis

    A. Nongonococcal urethritis.

B. Urinary tract infection.

C. Acute abdominal disorder in females with salpingitis.

D. Nongonococcal prostatitis.

VI. Prevention

A. Counsel patients (male or female) on use of condoms.

B. Counsel concerning early treatment of recurrence or reinfection.

C. Counsel on necessity of contact information in order to prevent further spread of the disease.

VII. Treatment

A. Patients for treatment

1. Patients with urethral discharge containing gram-negative intracellular and extracellular diplococci.

2. Patients with known recent exposure to gonorrhea.

3. Patients with positive cultures.

B. Drugs (for uncomplicated vaginitis or urethritis*):

1. Therapy of choice:

   a. Probenecid, 1 gm orally with aqueous procaine penicillin, 4.8 million units IM.

   or

   b. Ampicillin, 3.5 mg p.o. with probenecid one gm.

   or

   c. Amoxicillin, 3.0 grams with probenecid one gm.

   or

   d. Tetracycline, 0.5 gm orally 4 times a day for 5 days.

2. Therapy for patients with penicillin allergy:

   a. Tetracycline as above.

   or

   b. Spectinomycin, 2 gm IM (preferred during pregnancy).

Note: Because it is occasionally difficult to differentiate between nongonococcal and gonococcal urethritis, many people believe tetracycline is the drug of choice. Tetracycline, however, has the drawback of not being effective in a single dose, thus requiring the patient to follow through with a full course of treatment.

*Based on recommendations of the Center for Disease Control, Atlanta, Ga., 1979.

C. Instructions to patient

1. Avoid sexual activity for 2 days.
2. Ask sexual contacts to come to clinic for diagnosis and treatment.

VIII. Complications

A. Associated complications

1. Urethral stricture.
2. Rectal stricture.
3. Sterility (infrequent).

B. Infections beyond site of primary infection

1. Monarticular septic arthritis.
2. Disseminated gonococcal infection manifested primarily as skin lesions.
3. Gonococcal endocarditis.

C. The reappearance of urethral discharge after several days' absence

IX. Consultation-referral

A. Pharyngitis.

B. Proctitis.

C. Acute abdominal disorder or salpingitis.

D. Tender, swollen adnexa.

E. Fever above 100°F.

F. Arthritis.

G. Disseminated gonococcal infection with skin lesions.

H. Endocarditis.

I. Recurrence or positive follow-up culture.

J. Suspicion of penicillinase-producing N. gonorrhea

X. Follow-up. Culture in 7–14 days.

A. Males. Urethral culture.

B. Females. Cervical and anal cultures.

XI. Contact and reporting

A. Contact and treat all sexual partners.

B. Report primary case to the health department in the patient's county of residence.

Nonspecific Urethritis (Nongonococcal Urethritis): Adult

I. **Definition.** Infection of the urethra not caused by *Neisseria gonorrhoeae.*

II. **Etiology.** *Chlamydia* is felt to be the cause in at least half the cases.* In the remainder, the cause has not been identified.

III. **Clinical features**

   A. **Symptoms**

   1. In contrast to gonococcal infections may have had 1–2 weeks of symptoms.

   2. Dysuria.

   3. Increased urinary frequency.

   B. **Signs.** Urethral discharge, which is usually not as copious as in gonorrhea and may initially be present only on arising in the morning. The discharge may be milky in appearance and not purulent; however, this condition may mimic gonorrhea, presenting with extreme dysuria and purulent discharge.

IV. **Laboratory studies**

   A. Gram stain does not reveal gram-negative diplococci.

   B. Gonococcus cannot be cultured.

V. **Differential diagnosis.** This syndrome must be differentiated from gonococcal urethritis. Although there are some clinical differences, the diagnosis must be established by laboratory findings. There also may be a mixed infection of gonococcus and chlamydia. In this case discharge may initially disappear following treatment with penicillin, only to reappear in several days, often in a less purulent form. The second infection, postgonococcal urethritis (PGU), is from chlamydia not affected by penicillin.

VI. **Treatment.** If gram stain does not reveal gram-negative intracellular diplococci, treat with tetracycline, 500 mg 4 times a day for 7 days, or doxycycline 0.1 gram p.o. b.i.d. for 7 days.

VII. **Complications**

   A. Usually, there are no complications.

   B. In a small percentage of patients with a gram stain on which no gram-negative intracellular diplococci are found, the culture will be positive.

VIII. **Consultation-referral.** Failure of urethritis to respond to tetracycline.

*King K. Holmes. Etiology of nongonococcal urethritis. *N. Engl. J. Med.* 292:1199–1205, 1975.

IX. Follow-up

A. Return visit if symptoms do not improve.

B. Return visit if culture is positive for *N. gonorrhoeae,* for follow-up culture for *N. gonorrhoeae.*

Acute Bacterial Prostatitis: Adult

I. Definition. Acute bacterial infection of the prostate gland.

II. Etiology. Usually, *Escherichia coli* or other gram-negative bacteria that frequently cause infections of genitourinary tract.

III. Clinical features

A. Symptoms

1. Local

a. Pain in the lower back and perineum, which may be referred into the inguinal area and testes.

b. Symptoms of urinary obstruction or cystitis, or both.

c. Tenesmus.

2. Systemic

a. Fever.

b. Nausea.

c. Malaise.

d. Painful sexual intercourse or loss of libido.

B. Signs

1. Extremely tender, enlarged prostate. Do not massage.

2. Sometimes, temperature above 101°F.

3. Sometimes, penile discharge that is usually murky white, but may be purulent.

IV. Laboratory studies

A. Urinalysis usually shows both white and red blood cells.

B. Urine culture may be positive.

C. Gram stain of spun sediment may reveal bacteria.

V. Differential diagnosis

A. Low back pain from muscle strain or chronic prostatitis.

B. Febrile syndromes (e.g., "flu" syndrome) associated with back ache.

VI. Treatment

A. **Antibiotic.** Begin treatment when diagnosis is made—do not wait for results of culture:

1. Tetracycline, 250–500 mg orally 4 times a day for 14 days.

or

2. Ampicillin, 500 mg orally 4 times a day for 10 days.

B. **General**

1. Analgesic for pain.

2. Sitz bath for 30 minutes 3 times a day.

VII. Complications

A. Chronic bacterial prostatitis.

B. Urinary retention.

VIII. Consultation-referral

A. No improvement in 3 days.

B. Recurrence.

C. Temperature above 100°F.

D. Patient with diabetes mellitus.

E. Tenderness or swelling of epididymus or testicle.

F. Urinary retention.

IX. Follow-up. Reculture in 3 weeks if initial culture was positive.

Chronic Prostatitis:Adult

I. **Definition.** A condition of chronic infection or inflammation and congestion of the prostate, or both; may be bacterial or nonbacterial.

II. **Etiology**

A. **Bacterial.** The gram-negative bacteria commonly associated with genitourinary infection. Rarely, gram-positive organisms, such as *Staphylococcus saprophyticus.*

B. **Nonbacterial.** Cultures may be negative because of an antibacterial agent in prostatic fluid, mycoplasma of chlamydia may be the responsible organism, or the architecture of the prostate makes recovering bacteria from the infected site difficult.

III. **Clinical features**

A. **Symptoms**

1. Early morning penile discharge.

2. Vague urinary discomfort, frequently at the termination of micturition.

3. Dull ache in the perineum, often radiating into the groin or testicles.

4. Diminution of libido.

5. Low back pain.

6. No fever.

B. Signs. The prostate is slightly tender and slightly enlarged; it may be asymmetrical or boggy. Normal landmarks are preserved.

IV. Laboratory Studies. The ideal material for study is prostatic fluid. If this material cannot be obtained, a urine specimen voided after prostatic massage is satisfactory. This sample is compared with a urine specimen collected before massage.

A. Bacterial

1. Prostatic fluid contains greater than 10 white blood cells per high-power field, and gram stain of fluid shows bacteria.

2. Urine obtained after prostatic massage should contain white blood cells and bacteria.

3. Culture of prostatic fluid or urine voided after prostatic massage should produce gram-negative bacteria or, rarely, gram positive organisms, such as *Staphylococcus saprophyticus.*

B. Nonbacterial

1. Urine or prostatic fluid contains more than 10 white blood cells per high-power field but no bacteria.

2. Culture of urine or prostatic fluid does not produce bacteria.

V. Differential diagnosis

A. Acute bacterial prostatitis.

B. Other causes of low back pain.

C. Diseases of the anus, fissure, hemorrhoids.

D. Prostatodynia.

VI. Treatment

A. Bacterial. Chronic bacterial prostatis does not respond to many drugs because of poor diffusion of the drug into prostatic fluid.

1. Antibiotics

a. Doxycycline, 100 mg twice a day for 2 weeks.

or

b. Trimethoprim and sulfamethoxazole combination, 2 tablets twice a day for 4 weeks.

c. Erythromycin, 250 mg 4 times a day for 2 weeks, is used for gram-positive organisms; because of high levels possible in the prostate, may have some action against gram-negative bacteria.

d. Carbenicillin may be most effective, but reports are few. Consult phyician for use.

2. General measures

a. Sitz baths, 2 or 3 times a day for 15–20 minutes.

b. Explain to patient that increased sexual activity may help reduce prostatic congestion.

c. Analgesic for pain.

B. Nonbacterial

1. General treatment. See **VI.A.2.**

2. Prostatic massage may relieve pain from congestion.

VII. Complications

A. Obstruction of urinary outflow.

B. Chronic pain in the back and groin.

VIII. Consultation-referral

A. Bacterial. Failure of infection to resolve after initial antibiotic course.

B. Nonbacterial. Failure of symptoms to resolve after prostatic massage.

C. Recurrence of any symptoms.

IX. Follow-up

A. Bacterial. Return in 4–6 weeks for repeat urinalysis and culture.

B. Nonbacterial. Return if symptoms persist.

Benign Prostatic Hypertrophy: Adult

I. Definition. Hyperplasia of the periurethral glands and fibromuscular stroma, with overall enlargement of the gland and compression of the true prostatic tissue.

II. Etiology. The cause of benign prostatic hypertrophy is unknown, but normal testes seem to be necessary for BPH to occur. The disorder occurs with aging of the male, with symptoms and obstruction developing in 20% of males over 50–60 years of age and progressing to 50% of males over 80.

III. Clinical Features

A. Symptoms

1. Difficulty in starting micturition.

2. Difficulty in stopping urine flow.

3. Small urinary stream.

4. Small amounts voided frequently.

5. Nocturia.

Note: Nocturia is an important finding and suggests that there have been changes in the bladder wall sufficient to cause post-void residual and frequently indicates the need for surgery.

B. Signs

1. Diffuse enlargement of the prostate gland is present.

2. No nodules are present. Normal landmarks are preserved.

3. Bladder may be palpable or percussible above the symphysis pubis if obstruction is present.

IV. Laboratory studies

A. Blood urea nitrogen and creatinine levels.

B. Urinalysis, including microscopic examination.

C. Urine culture (clean-catch urine specimen).

V. Differential diagnosis

A. Other causes of obstruction to urinary flow, particularly urethral stricture.

B. Carcinoma of the prostate.

C. Inflammation of the prostate.

D. Other causes of nocturia, such as diabetes and congestive heart failure.

Note: In diabetes and congestive heart failure, patients pass large volumes of urine. In benign prostatic hypertrophy, there is frequent, difficult voiding of small amounts of urine.

VI. Treatment.
There is no medical treatment for benign prostatic hypertrophy. When symptoms of obstruction occur, the patient must be referred to a urologist for surgical therapy. Because of the prevalence of this disease in elderly males, one must be aware of the potential complications of an enlarged prostate.

VII. Complications

A. Increasing obstruction.

B. Secondary infection.

C. Renal failure.

D. Congestive heart failure.

Note: In patients with compromised cardiac function, the inability to pass sufficient urine can lead to fluid retention and congestive heart failure.

VIII. Consultation-referral

A. Significant symptoms of obstruction or a palpable or percussible bladder, or both.

B. Nocturia of 2–3 times a night.

C. Acute or symptomatic infection of prostate, or both.

D. Laboratory evidence of decreased renal function.

E. Recurrent urinary tract infection.

IX. Follow-up.
Obtain history related to voiding at least once a year, or every visit, if visits occur less frequently than once a year. Also, do rectal examination annually.

Vulvovaginitis: Pediatric

I. Definition. Inflammation of the vulva and vagina, commonly presenting with discharge, pruritus, and erythema.

II. Etiology*

A. Nonspecific origin. This type of vulvovaginitis is usually associated with poor hygiene, and no specific microorganism is incriminated. Culture reveals mixed flora of colonic bacteria (the most common cause in prepubertal females). The inflammation may be aggravated by tight undergarments, especially panty hose or leotards.

B. Irritant

1. Bubble bath (relatively common).

2. Foreign body in vagina (often, wads of toilet paper not palpable on rectal examination). Bloody, purulent discharge may ensue.

*For any complaints related to the genital area, the examiner should explore the possibility of sexual abuse.

C. Bacteria

1. Group A beta-hemolytic streptococci (occasionally associated with scarlet fever).

2. Gonococcus, causing vaginitis in prepubertal females and endocervicitis in older females. In prepubertal patients, gonococcal infection strongly indicates sexual abuse.

3. Other oganisms, including *Staphylococcus aureus* (labial abscess or impetigo causing vulvitis) and *Gardnerella vaginalis* (more common in older females).

D. Parasites

1. Pinworms, which move from the anus into the vagina, where they cause mechanical irritation and scratching.

2. *Trichomonas vaginalis* common *after* puberty; prepubertal strongly indicates sexual abuse.

E. Fungus. Vulvovaginitis due to *Candida albicans* is common after puberty but occasionally is seen in very young infants, where spread is by hands from vaginitis in an adult.

F. Virus

1. Herpesvirus hominis type 2 usually causes infection in the postpubertal period; see Chapter 3, Herpes Simplex (Pediatric and Adult).

2. Vulvovaginitis may be associated with measles or varicella.

III. Clinical features

A. Symptoms

1. Pruritus.

2. Vaginal discharge.

3. Dysuria.

4. Enuresis.

5. Pain with walking or sitting.

6. In a younger child, awkward motions, keeping thighs together while moving, or scratching.

B. Signs

1. Vaginal discharge is usually purulent, and occasionally blood-tinged if a foreign body is present.

2. Excoriations may be present.

3. Erythema of vulva may be present.

4. If hygiene is poor, one may see either bits of stool in the perineal area or pasty, white material between the labial grooves.

5. A foreign body, if hard, may be felt on compression of the vagina during rectal examination.

IV. Laboratory studies

A. Smear of vaginal discharge

1. Obtain a fresh specimen with a cotton swab or dropper after cleansing the vulva.

2. Wet preparation with saline is used to identify *Trichomonas* organisms.

3. Wet preparation with potassium hydroxide is used to detect *Candida* budding yeast with or without hyphae.

4. Gram stain results are sometimes difficult to interpret because of the large variety of organisms found in the normal prepubertal vagina. Gram stain is also unreliable for diagnosing gonococcal infection because of the similar appearance of some nonpathogenic organisms.

B. Culture of vulval and vaginal secretions

1. Obtain vaginal specimen by inserting a moist sterile cotton swab after culturing and cleansing the vulva.

2. Order routine bacterial culture.

3. Order gonococcal culture.

Note: The normal prepuberal vagina has a great variety of nonpathogenic bacteria, including *Escherichia coli, Klebsiella,* enterococci, alpha streptococci, *Staphylococcus epidermidis, Proteus,* diphtheroids, *Lactobacillus,* and *Pseudomonas.*

V. Differential diagnosis

A. Discharge seen normally in first 2 weeks of life (white, nonpurulent, nonodorous, and nonirritating).

B. Discharge seen normally in pubertal and immediate prepubertal period (asymptomatic and white or mucoid).

VI. Treatment. Treatment is specific, depending on etiology:

A. Patient should discontinue bubble bath.

B. Treat for pinworms if they are seen by a reliable observer (see Chapter 15, Pinworms [Pediatric and Adult], **VI,** p. 342), but **consult also** because of the possibility of trapped vaginal pinworms.

C. Treat for specific pathogenic bacteria after review of culture results and clinical evidence with consultant.

D. See guidelines in Chapter 14 for **candidal vaginitis** and **trichomonal vaginitis** in postpubertal patients. Because *Trichomonas* may be transmitted venereally, counsel patient appropriately.

E. Use the following measures for **nonspecific vulvovaginitis** and as **general treatment** for all patients:

1. **Perineal hygiene.** Instruct patient in the following hygiene practices:

   a. Bathe the perineum gently but carefully with warm water and nonperfumed, nonmedicated soap twice a day and after defecation.

   b. Remove smegma from between interlabial grooves.

   c. Blot dry—do not rub with a towel.

   d. Then air-dry, with perineum exposed to warm, dry air.

   e. Wear loose, clean, absorbent (cotton) underpants, and change them frequently. Do not wear panty hose or leotards.

   f. After defecation, wipe from front to back, with hand coming from behind.

   g. Educate child about perineal hygiene if she is old enough. Have mother observe child practicing.

2. **Sitz baths.** Patient should take a daily sitz bath with an acidifying solution (2 tablespoons of vinegar per quart of warm water) to make the vulval and vaginal mucosa less favorable for bacterial growth and to provide symptomatic relief.

3. **Cold compresses.** If the vulva is very edematous and tender, patient can apply cold compresses of tap water or aluminum acetate (Borow's) solution for 20 minutes 4 times a day.

VII. Complications. Irritation of the perineum, with development of dermatitis and secondary bacterial skin infection.

VIII. Consultation-referral

A. Clinical or laboratory evidence of a bacterial pathogen. Review bacterial culture results with the physician if the organisms are not listed as nonpathogenic in **IV.B. Note.**

B. Pinworm infestation and vulvovaginitis.

C. Suspicion of a foreign body.

D. Failure to respond to treatment within 1 week. These patients will probably need vaginoscopy to rule out a foreign body.

E. *Trichomonas vaginalis* in prepubertal child.

F. Any case in which sexual molestation is a possibility.

IX. **Follow-up.** Return visit in 1 week or sooner if results of culture indicate a need for additional therapy.

Enuresis: Pediatric

I. **Definition.** An involuntary passage of urine during the day or night. Nocturnal enuresis occurs in about 10–15% of 5-year-olds, 5% of 10-year-olds, and 1% of 15-year-olds.

II. **Etiology**

   A. **Unknown cause.** This is the most common category. Numerous etiologic theories have been advanced; however, there is no unanimous agreement among authorities. These theories include:

   1. Psychologic factors.

   2. Limited bladder capacity.

   3. Delayed neurologic maturation.

   4. Profound sleep state.

   B. **Variation of normal.** Under 5 years of age, enuresis can be considered normal unless there are signs and symptoms suggesting a specific cause.

   C. **Urinary tract infection**

   D. **Obstructive lesions of the urinary tract**

   E. **Primary neurologic disorder**

   F. Disorders associated with **decreased urine-concentrating ability and increased volume,** causing enuresis.

III. **Clinical features**

   A. **Symptoms**

   1. The passage of urine may occur from rarely to several times daily, day or night. In children who have achieved good control, there may be periodic lapses at night for several years.

   2. Boys are affected somewhat more frequently than girls.

   3. There is a familial tendency.

   B. **Signs.** Results of a complete physical examination are usually normal; however, particular attention should be paid to:

   1. Evidence of psychologic and behavior problems.

   2. Lumbosacral skin abnormalities.

   3. Abnormalities of the genitalia, including the urethral meatus.

4. Poor rectal sphincter tone.

5. Decreased perineal sensation to pinprick.

IV. Laboratory studies

A. Urinalysis and measurement of specific gravity (ideally on a first morning specimen to assess concentrating ability).

B. Urine culture; see Urinary Tract Infection (Pediatric), **IV.A,** p. 230, for technique and interpretation.

V. Differential diagnosis. None.

VI. Treatment

A. General counseling

1. If child is under 5 years of age, reassure that enuresis is still normal at that age unless symptoms or signs suggest a specific cause.

2. Advise parents not to ridicule or punish for enuresis, as it is not voluntary. Secondary psychologic problems can result if enuresis is managed inappropriately by the family.

3. Reassure that even if nothing is done, enuresis is most often a self-limiting condition if there is no specific underlying cause that can be found.

B. Therapy for children over 5 years of age (after examination and laboratory studies reveal no specific cause)

1. Have patient keep a diary of wet and dry days and nights for 1 month.

2. If daytime enuresis occurs, consult physician.

3. If only nocturnal enuresis occurs, suggest the following measures (the efficacy of these suggestions has not been proved, but each has the support of some clinicians):

   a. Limit fluid intake after evening meal and have child urinate before going to bed.

   b. Suggest that before the parents go to bed, they awaken the child to urinate.

   c. Encourage the child to become involved in the therapeutic process:

   (1) Have the patient keep a diary of wet and dry nights.

   (2) Have parents give praise and small rewards for dry nights.

   (3) Suggest that the patient retain urine for progressively longer periods during the day.

     d. Schedule return visit in 1 month.

     e. If enuresis has not decreased, consult the physician.

     f. If enuresis has decreased, give praise and continue to see the patient periodically on the basis of degree of improvement and need for counseling.

    4. Punishment or ridicule by family should be strictly prohibited.

VII. Complications. Secondary psychologic problems because of:

    A. Punitive or ridiculing family attitude.

    B. Inability of child to participate in certain social activities, such as camp and overnight visits.

VIII. Consultation-referral

    A. Daytime enuresis.

    B. Evidence suggesting specific organic cause.

    C. Severe psychologic problems.

    D. Failure to improve after treatment.

IX. Follow-up. See **IV.B.3.d–f.**

Urinary Incontinence: Adult

I. Definition. Involuntary passage of urine that is a social or hygienic problem for the patient.

II. Etiology. Urination occurs when pressure within the bladder overcomes resistance of the sphincter. Bladder and sphincter tone is maintained by a complex neurologic system that extends from cortical centers through the spinal column to the bladder detrusor muscles. Sphincter competence is further supported by estrogen effects on the urethral mucosa and by the urethro-vesicular angle.

    A. Instability of the detrusor muscle (spastic bladder). Bladder contractions overcome normal sphincter tone. May cause more than 70% of incontinence in the elderly.

    B. Overflow incontinence (incontinence at very high bladder volumes). Associated with bladder outlet obstruction, decreased bladder tone, and decreased bladder sensation.

    C. Stress incontinence. (Decreased sphincter competence.) Besides neuromuscular structures, sphincter competence is maintained by estrogen effects on the urethral mucosa and maintenance of vesico-urethral angle.

    D. Functional incontinence related to other medical conditions, fecal impaction, urinary infection, medications, or altered mental status.

III. Clinical features

  A. Symptoms. Workup should include a detailed history of the pattern of incontinence, including precipitants, past history of urologic and neurologic disease, and medications.

    1. Patients with destrusor instability may have a sensation of bladder fullness or urgency with little warning before passage of urine.

    2. Overflow incontinence is manifested by frequent loss of small amounts of urine.

    3. Stress incontinence may be precipitated by coughing, laughing, or later, by simply rising from a chair.

    4. Functional incontinence may occur in the setting of a progressive dementing illness, sedating medication, or in association with diminished communication or motor function after a CVA.

  B. Physical examination

    1. Neurologic examination including mental status.

    2. Abdominal and pelvic examination for evidence of a distended bladder, cystocele, or atrophic vaginitis (secondary to estrogen deficiency).

    3. Test for perineal sensation including anal sphincter tone.

    4. Rectal examination to rule out fecal impaction or prostatic disease.

    5. Assessment of functional ability to carry out a complete urinary maneuver.

    6. Other assessments may be indicated by deterioration in general condition.

IV. Diagnostic and laboratory studies

  A. Urinalysis for evidence of infection; blood glucose, BUN, calcium.

  B. Catheterization for post-void residual urine.

  C. The above tests are sufficient for initial evaluation. Some patients may need further tests following consultation, particularly patients found to have obstruction, overflow, or stress incontinence. These patients may benefit from studies which include an IVP, cystoscopy, or urodynamic measurements.

V. Conditions associated with incontinence

A. Fecal impaction.

B. Urinary tract infection.

C. Medication effect (diuretics, sedatives).

D. Atrophic vaginitis.

E. A variety of neurologic diseases, including spinal cord lesions. The simultaneous occurrence of urinary and fecal incontinence is suspicious for a spinal cord lesion.

VI. Treatment. The above conditions should be treated. If incontinence remains, consultation is required. Many, perhaps most of the remaining cases of urinary incontinence in the elderly can be successfully treated, however, especially if intervention is begun soon after symptoms appear. Treatment is specific to the type of incontinence found. Plans of care should be developed after physician consultation and must anticipate multiple trials of therapy. Diapering or permanent indwelling catheters represent failures of medical treatment.

VII. Complications

A. Social isolation of the patient and frustration for the family.

B. Skin breakdown.

VIII. Consultation-referral

A. All cases of new-onset urinary incontinence require physician consultation once fecal impaction and urinary infection have been ruled out and a careful medication review has been performed.

IX. Follow-up. Therapy of urinary incontinence may require therapeutic trials or a number of medications or behavioral interventions. Frequent follow-up is necessary after every intervention, and supportive contact with family is helpful.

Disorders of the Musculoskeletal System

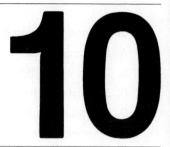

Minor Ankle Sprain: Pediatric and Adult

I. **Definition.** An injury to the ankle resulting in stretching of the ligament. In a mild sprain, there is no tear of the ligament.

II. **Etiology.** Sprain is most often due to inversion-plantar flexion injury ("I turned my ankle").

III. **Clinical features**

    A. **Symptoms**

        1. Pain over the lateral aspect of the ankle.

        2. Patient did *not* hear or feel a "pop" or "snap" at the time of injury (these suggest a ligamental tear or fracture).

    B. **Signs**

        1. *No* ecchymoses.

        2. Minimal, somewhat diffuse tenderness over the medial or lateral malleolus.

        3. *No* focal area of exquisite tenderness.

        4. Minimal or *no* swelling.

        5. No instability of joint.

IV. **Diagnostic studies.** With mild injury, x-ray films are not indicated.

V. **Differential diagnosis**

    A. Ligamental tears.

    B. Fractures.

VI. **Treatment**

    A. Tell patient to keep weight off the ankle, with either bed rest or use of crutches.

    B. Wrap ankle with Ace bandage.

C. An ice pack may be applied to the ankle for the first 24 hours to prevent swelling.

D. Follow with heat to the ankle, if necessary.

E. Aspirin (325 mg per tablet), 2 tablets orally 4 times a day, for analgesic and anti-inflammatory effects for adults.

or

F. In case of intolerance to aspirin in adults, acetaminophen (325 mg per tablet), 2 tablets orally 4 times a day. For pediatric dosage, see p. 151.

VII. **Complications.** None with minor sprain.

VIII. **Consultation-referral**

A. All sprains associated with ecchymoses, focal or moderate to severe tenderness, more than minimal swelling, or instability of a joint.

B. All possible fractures.

IX. **Follow-up.** Return visit in 24 hours; if the sprain is not significantly improved, refer for x-ray study and consultation.

Minor Strains and Sprains*: Pediatric and Adult

I. **Definition.** Minor injury to a joint where the nature of the trauma was mild, resulting in minimal stretching of the involved ligaments and contusion of the surrounding soft tissues.

II. **Etiology.** Strains and sprains usually result from a fall, a blow from another person, or an automobile accident. In cases to be managed by the nurse practitioner, the history of the nature of the injury should suggest only minor trauma; for example, falling on the ground, a child's receiving a blow from another child, or a minor automobile accident. Although minor trauma does not ensure that the injury is not severe, it is an important point to notice. All cases involving major trauma, such as severe automobile accidents, should *not* be managed by the nurse practitioner.

III. **Clinical features**

A. **Symptoms**

1. Mild pain around the site of injury.

2. Minimal or no loss of function of the involved area.

*Excluding ankle sprains. For these, see Minor Ankle Sprain (Pediatric and Adult), p. 252.

B. Signs

1. No ecchymoses.
2. No instability.
3. No focal tenderness over the involved ligaments or bones.
4. No crepitance.
5. *Minimal* or *no* swelling of the involved area.

IV. Diagnostic studies. X-ray films are not indicated in minor injuries.

V. Differential diagnosis

A. Severe sprain with or without fracture, suggested by these symptoms:

1. Severe pain.
2. Loss of function.
3. Ecchymoses.
4. Point tenderness.
5. Instability.
6. Crepitance.
7. Moderate or severe swelling.

B. Fractures.

VI. Treatment

A. Immobilization of joint for 24–36 hours.

B. Ice pack for 24 hours.

C. Local heat after first 24 hours, if needed.

D. Aspirin (325 mg per tablet), 2 tablets orally 4 times a day, for analgesic and anti-inflammatory effects for adults.

or

E. In case of intolerance to aspirin in adults, acetaminophen (325 mg tablets), 2 orally 4 times a day. For pediatric dosage, see p. 151.

or

F. Ibuprofen (Motrin®) 400 mg orally 4 times a day.

VII. Complications. None.

VIII. Consultation-referral. All injuries associated with:

A. Ecchymoses.

B. Focal or moderate to severe tenderness.

C. More than minimal swelling.

D. Instability of the joint.

IX. Follow-up. A return visit is mandatory if there is *no* improvement in 24 hours or incomplete resolution in 1 week.

Musculoskeletal Chest Pain: Adult

I. Definition. Pain in the chest arising from (1) the bony structures of the rib cage and associated upper-limb girdle, (2) the skeletal muscle related to the chest and upper limb, or (3) a combination of these.

II. Etiology. The pain frequently is related to unusual muscular exertion involving the upper limb or chest, or both. Trauma may be implicated. In many cases, the cause is unknown.

III. Clinical features

A. Symptoms

1. The pain is usually aggravated by activity producing either movement of the chest cage or upper extremity or pressure on the chest, or both, and is relieved by rest or release of pressure.

2. The pain is *not produced by general exertion,* such as walking up a flight of stairs, or other exertion not requiring movement of the chest or arm.

3. The pain often occurs late in the day after the patient has indulged in strenuous exertion involving the chest or arm.

4. The pain is frequently described as sharp, momentary, and stabbing.

B. Signs

1. Pain is often reproduced by either movement of the arm or chest or pressure on the chest cage or muscles involved, or both.

2. The chest is clear on auscultation.

3. Cardiac examination is normal.

IV. Diagnostic studies

A. Seldom indicated.

B. Electrocardiography may be done in older patients for reassurance. One should not rely on the electrocardiogram to make a diagnosis, however.

V. Differential diagnosis

A. Angina pectoris.

B. Myocardial infarction.

   C. Pleuritic chest pain.

   D. Esophagitis and other gastrointestinal causes of chest pain.

   E. Cervical spine disease (disc disease and osteophytosis produce nerve root compression).

VI. Treatment

   A. Reassure patient as to the origin of the pain.

   B. Advise patient on these measures:

      1. Heat to the involved area.

      2. Rest.

      3. Aspirin (325 mg per tablet), 2 tablets orally every 4–6 hours; acetaminophen (325 mg per tablet), 2 tablets orally every 4–6 hours; or Ibuprofen (Motrin®) 400 mg orally 4 times a day.

VII. Complications. These are primarily psychologic, relating to the patient's concern that the pain is cardiac in origin.

VIII. Consultation-referral

   A. Unclear diagnosis.

   B. Unusual patient anxiety, even if the diagnosis seems readily apparent.

IX. Follow-up. As needed to reassure both the patient and the nurse practitioner.

Lumbosacral Strain: Adult

   I. Definition. A painful condition involving the lower back. It is usually recurrent, with acute exacerbations often related to physical stress (80% of adults will develop back pain at some time).

   II. Etiology. Pain arises from strain of the ligaments and musculature of the lumbosacral area, and not from the vertebrae, articular cartilage, or nerve roots.

  III. Clinical features

   A. Symptoms

      1. Usually mild to moderately severe pain located across the lumbosacral area, generally worsened by movement, such as getting out of bed, rising from a sitting position, or bending over.

      2. No radicular pain.

      3. No radiation of pain to legs, groin, or testes.

      4. No costovertebral angle pain.

    5. No dysuria, frequency, or other genitourinary symptoms.

    6. No bladder or bowel incontinence.

B. Signs

    1. No fever.

    2. Pain and muscle spasm on palpation over lumbosacral area may be present.

    3. No pain in flanks on percussion.

    4. Straight leg-raising should not produce pain that radiates down the leg.

    5. Normal neurologic examination of lower extremities, including sensory and motor function and reflexes.

    6. Intact pulses in lower extremities.

IV. Diagnostic studies. None.

V. Differential diagnosis

    A. Lumbosacral disc disease.

    B. Genitourinary infections, including cystitis, prostatitis, and pyelonephritis.

    C. Vascular occlusion at the level of the aortic bifurcation.

    D. Cancer with bony metastases (cancer of the prostate often presents in this manner).

    E. Gynecologic disorders (e.g., endometriosis and fibromyomas).

VI. Treatment. Advise patient on these measures:

    A. Education about back care.

    B. For moderately severe pain, bed rest. For minimal pain, restriction of activity, particularly lifting.

    C. Bed board.

    D. Local heat.

    E. Back flexion exercises.

    F. Aspirin (325 mg per tablet), 2 tablets orally 4 times a day.

    or

    G. In case of intolerance to aspirin, acetaminophen (325 mg tablets), 2 orally 4 times a day.

    or

    H. Ibuprofen (Motrin®), 400 mg orally four times a day.

VII. **Complications.** Prolonged disability that is probably due to a combination of physical, psychologic, social, and economic factors.

VIII. **Consultation-referral**

   A. Severe, disabling pain.

   B. Prolonged pain (lasting more than 2 weeks).

   C. Recurrent pain (more than three attacks).

   D. Neurologic deficit (motor or sensory).

   E. Bladder or bowel incontinence, which may indicate involvement of autonomic nerves.

IX. **Follow-up.** Return visit if there is no improvement within several days.

Nonspecific Musculoskeletal Pain: Adult

   I. **Definition.** Vague aching of the muscles, bones, joints, or ligaments (alone or in any combination), usually poorly localized to areas such as the arm and shoulder, the hip and leg, and the anterior chest and arm.

   II. **Etiology**

   A. Trauma or straining of the involved area by excessive use is often implicated.

   B. Frequently, no obvious cause can be ascertained.

   C. Nonspecific musculoskeletal pain is often associated with tension-anxiety states.

   III. **Clinical features**

   A. **Symptoms**

      1. A vague aching of the muscles, bones, joints, or ligaments, usually poorly localized to areas such as the arm and shoulder, the hip and leg, and the anterior chest and arm.

      2. *No* generalized myalgia.

      3. *No* localized musculoskeletal pain, as in bursitis or arthritis.

      4. *No* neurologic symptoms, such as sensory loss or localized weakness.

      5. Sometimes, history of trauma to or excessive or unusual use of the involved area.

   B. **Signs**

      1. No fever.

  2. No objective inflammation, that is, no redness, swelling, heat, or warmth of any part of the painful area.

  3. No demonstrable sensory or motor deficit.

  4. Sometimes, vague, poorly localized tenderness to palpation of the involved muscles, joints, ligaments, or bones.

IV. Diagnostic studies. None.

V. Differential diagnosis

  A. Specific localized inflammatory conditions affecting the musculoskeletal system (e.g., arthritis, bursitis, tendinitis, and gout).

  B. Generalized myalgia accompanying systemic illnesses (e.g., influenza, Rocky Mountain spotted fever, and pneumonia).

  C. Specific localized symptoms related to known trauma (e.g., sprained ankle).

VI. Treatment. Advise patient on these measures:

  A. Rest of the involved area.

  B. Heat by means of a hot water bottle, heating pad, warm soaks, hot showers, etc.

  C. Aspirin (325 mg per tablet), 2 tablets orally 4 times a day.

  or

  D. In case of intolerance to aspirin, acetaminophen (325 mg per tablet), 2 orally 4 times a day.

  or

  E. Ibuprofen (Motrin®), 400 mg orally four times a day.

VII. Complications. Prolonged disability.

VIII. Consultation-referral

  A. Severe pain.

  B. Course prolonged more than 2 weeks.

  C. Recurrent pain (more than three attacks).

IX. Follow-up. As needed.

Degenerative Joint Disease (Osteoarthritis): Adult

  I. Definition. A disorder usually restricted to elderly people and characterized by degeneration of articular cartilage and hypertrophy of bone, usually in weight-bearing joints and in the distal interphalangeal joints of the fingers.

II. Etiology. Degenerative joint disease is associated with aging and trauma, but no specific cause has been found.

III. Clinical features

A. Symptoms

1. Joint pain and stiffness are present. The pain characteristically improves with rest and worsens with exercise, while the stiffness improves with exercise.

2. Pain is usually mild and rarely progresses to the point of invalidism, although it may become difficult to move the affected fingers easily and with precision.

3. Cervical lesions may lead to neck pain and may cause radicular neuropathy, with pain and weakness in the arm or the shoulder girdle.

B. Signs

1. The joints most commonly affected are the knees, hips, lumbar vertebrae (weight-bearing joints), cervical vertebrae, and distal interphalangeal joints of the fingers.

2. Affected joints are not hot or erythematous, but may be mildly tender.

3. Classically, interphalangeal involvement leads to Heberden's nodes—firm, knotty enlargements of the distal interphalangeal joints—which may be present alone without other joint involvement.

4. Larger joints and vertebrae usually appear grossly normal.

IV. Laboratory and other studies

A. An x-ray film of the involved joint is useful if the diagnosis is in question (Heberden's nodes do not require x-ray).

B. Determination of the sedimentation rate also may be helpful to establish the presence or absence of an inflammatory process. Should be normal in degenerative joint disease.

V. Differential diagnosis

A. Polyarthritis

1. Acute rheumatoid arthritis is usually easily differentiated because the affected joints are inflamed, there may be constitutional signs and symptoms, the sedimentation rate is elevated, and it occurs less frequently in elderly people.

2. Chronic rheumatoid arthritis affects the proximal interphalangeal and the metacarpo-phalangeal joints.

3. In addition to bone involvement, there is swelling of synovial tissue and edema around the joints in both acute and chronic rheumatoid arthritis.

B. Monarticular arthritis

1. Gout (see Chapter 12, Gout and Hyperuricemia [Adult], pp. 286–290).

2. Traumatic arthritis. Generally, the joints are swollen and tender, and there is a history of trauma.

3. Infection. Inflammatory arthritis is frequently associated with gonococcal infection occurring in a much younger age group.

Note: Osteoarthritis may be present along with an inflammatory arthritis. If the degree of pain and inflammation seems incompatible with osteoarthritis, one should seek another cause.

VI. Treatment. Advise patient on these measures:

A. Rest of the involved joints.

B. Physical therapy of the joints.

C. Aspirin or acetaminophen (325 mg) for pain—2 tablets orally every 4–6 hours, or Ibuprofen (Motrin®), 400 mg orally four times a day.

D. Heat to the involved joints.

E. Weight loss and elimination of trauma.

F. In some cases, a neck or back support.

VII. Complications

A. Generally, osteoarthritis is not severe or crippling and usually results in no systemic complaints.

B. Cervical vertebral lesions occasionally lead to radicular neurologic problems.

VIII. Consultation-referral

A. Inflammatory arthritis.

B. Neurologic involvement.

IX. Follow-up

A. These patients may be seen as needed for exacerbation of pain or dysfunction.

B. Special visits generally are not necessary; the osteoarthritis may be evaluated during visits for other problems or for health maintenance.

Osteoporosis: Adult

I. **Definition.** A heterogeneous group of diseases resulting in a reduction in bone mass per unit volume below the level required for adequate mechanical support. The ratio of mineral to matrix material remains normal. This reduction may ultimately lead to fractures.

II. **Etiology.** Multiple known causes for osteoporosis include corticosteroid therapy, chronic heparin therapy, prolonged immobilization, and calcium deficiency. Most cases, however, are of unclear etiology. The risk of osteoporosis increases with age, female sex, white race, and menopause, especially secondary to surgical removal of the ovaries.

III. **Clinical features**

A. **Symptoms**

1. Most patients are asymptomatic as they undergo slow reduction in their bone density.

2. Back pain related to vertebral compression fractures is the most common symptomatic presentation.

3. Fracture of the hip may be the first indication of significant bone disease.

B. **Physical examination**

1. May have no physical signs.

2. Kyphosis.

3. Loss of height.

IV. **Laboratory and diagnostic studies**

A. X-rays may show decreased bone density, but this may be evident only after > 40% of bony mass is lost.

B. Bone densitometry may detect early bone loss, but its precise role in diagnosis is unclear.

C. Complete blood count, calcium, and alkaline phosphatase should be obtained, but will be normal in idiopathic osteoporosis.

V. **Differential diagnosis**

A. Vitamin D deficiency.

B. Metastatic carcinoma.

C. Multiple myeloma.

D. Cortisol excess, either intrinsic (Cushing's disease) or from use of exogenous steroids.

E. Osteoarthritis may cause back pain, but has a very different clinical course and x-ray picture.

VI. Treatment

A. Prevention. Primary prevention of bone loss seems to be more effective in preventing symptoms than treatment after pain or fractures have occurred.

1. Women who have undergone premature surgical oophorectomy should receive estrogen replacement.

2. Estrogen replacement in women at the time of physiologic menopause may be indicated in women at risk for fractures (white race, thin body habitus, family history of fractures).

3. Maintenance of an adequate calcium intake (greater than 1.0 gram elemental calcium per day) may have some protective effect, and is unlikely to do harm. This addition may be in the form of increased intake of dairy products or use of over-the-counter calcium supplements. Such dietary supplementation, when administered, should begin well before menopause. After menopause, some authors recommend 1.5 grams of elemental calcium per day. The utility of supplemental vitamin D in patients with adequate natural intake is controversial.

4. Maintenance of moderate physical activity with aging may preserve bony mass.

Note: Use of conjugated estrogens has been linked with later development of endometrial cancer. When this class of medications is administered to a patient with a uterus, the patient should be informed of the risks, and appropriate consultation obtained about follow-up. Risk of endometrial carcinoma may in theory be decreased by cycling estrogens 21 out of 28 days and by using progestational agents.

VII. Complications

A. Fracture of the femoral neck with mild or minimal trauma.

B. Other fractures, including vertebral compression fractures.

VIII. Consultation-referral

A. All patients being considered for estrogen therapy require consultation.

B. Consultation for all patients with symptomatic back pain related to compression fractures.

IX. Follow-up

A. Preventive interventions should be addressed at health care maintenance visits.

B. Follow-up for symptomatic patients should be individualized.

Disorders of the Nervous System

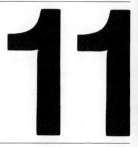

Dizziness in Adults Less Than Fifty Years Old

I. **Definition.** A vague sensation of unsteadiness or lightheadedness, or both, occurring episodically in adults less than 50 years old. This is a common complaint in all ages, but in the young adult most often is inconsequential and must be differentiated from the problems below.

II. **Etiology.** Most often seen in association with tension-anxiety states.

III. **Clinical features**

  A. **Symptoms**

    1. A vague sensation of unsteadiness, as though one might fall in one direction or another.

    2. No vertigo.

    3. No tendency to fall consistently in one direction.

    4. No associated severe headache.

    5. No associated neurologic symptoms.

    6. No associated nausea or vomiting.

    7. Feeling of faintness or sensation of loss of consciousness, but no actual loss of consciousness.

    8. Attacks are neither precipitated by prior ingestion (1–1½ hours before attack) of heavy carbohydrate meal nor relieved by ingestion of food.

  B. **Signs**

    1. Blood pressure between 100/70 and 150/100 mm Hg, with orthostatic drop of less than 10 mg Hg diastolic.

    2. Normal neurologic examination.

    3. No murmur of aortic stenosis.

IV. **Laboratory studies.** Hematocrit or hemoglobin or both are normal.

V. Differential diagnosis

A. Vasovagal syncope.

B. Vertiginous dizziness, as in labyrinthitis, Ménière's disease, and acoustic neuroma.

C. Postural hypotension, especially in patients being treated for hypertension.

D. Acute blood loss, as in gastrointestinal hemorrhage.

E. Unsteadiness associated with significant anemia (hematocrit reading less than 35%).

F. Dizziness associated with aortic stenosis.

G. Dizziness associated with other neurologic symptoms or signs, as in a stroke syndrome.

H. Hypoglycemic episodes.

VI. Treatment

A. Reassure patient as to the absence of serious disease.

B. Attempt to discover and alter psychosocial factors that often are associated.

VII. Complications. Prolonged disability.

VIII. Consultation-referral. Severe, persistent (single attack lasting more than 24 hours), or recurring (more than six per week) attacks.

IX. Follow-up. As needed.

Migraine Headache: Adult

I. Definition. A throbbing unilateral headache with familial tendency that is preceded by an aura and by other neurologic manifestations in many cases.

II. Etiology. Unknown. Pain is related to cerebral arterial spasm followed by dilation. It is during the dilation phase that pain occurs.

III. Clinical features

A. Headache is usually unilateral, but not always on the same side.

B. Headaches are generally preceded by a visual aura, which may be followed by neurologic signs, such as tingling and weakness in an extremity. There may actually be temporary paralysis.

C. Throbbing gradually increases in intensity to a peak in 1 hour and then may last for a few hours to several days. It may be associated with nausea and vomiting.

D. Photophobia may be present.

E. Eighty percent of patients have a family history of migraine.

F. Onset is usually in adolescence, and attacks tend to decrease in frequency with age. Migraine may, however, begin at a later age and actually accelerate in frequency during menopause.

IV. Laboratory studies. None.

V. Differential diagnosis. See Tension Headache (Adult), **V**, p. 268.

VI. Treatment

A. Patient can use either of the following at the first sign of headache:

1. Ergotamine tartrate (Ergostat)—2 mg sublingually initially, followed by 2 mg every hour until headache is relieved, to a maximum of 6 mg per day or 10 mg per week.

    or

2. A combination of 1 mg ergotamine tartrate and 100 mg caffeine (Cafergot)—2 tablets orally initially, followed by 1 tablet every hour until headache is relieved, to a maximum of 6 tablets per day or 10 tablets per week. This may also be taken as a rectal suppository—(2 mg ergotamine tartrate and 100 mg caffeine), 1 suppository initially, followed by 1 suppository in an hour if needed (maximum, 2 per day)—if vomiting precludes oral administration.

    Note: Ergotamine tartrate is contraindicated in moderate to severe hypertension, vascular diseases, renal disease, and pregnancy.

B. In established headache, an ergot preparation may be tried (see **A**), but generally the following measures are required:

1. Dark room

2. Analgesic, such as codeine or meperidine HCl (Demerol). Both are controlled medicines requiring physician's orders.

C. One of the following may be used as preventive therapy under a physician's direction to decrease the frequency of attacks:

1. Bellergal (often effective when there seems to be a psychologic overlay to the problem).

2. Propranolol HCl (Inderal).

3. Methysergide maleate (Sansert).

4. Tricyclic antidepressants.

VII. Complications. Generally, there are no complications.

VIII. Consultation-referral

    A. Failure of treatment.

    B. All new cases (first time to clinic or first time with headache).

    C. Persistence of neurologic component.

  IX. Follow-up. Return visit if there is no improvement.

Tension Headache: Adult

  I. Definition. A headache that is generally associated with periods of stress and is characterized by bandlike pressure across the forehead and occiput.

  II. Etiology. The headache is generally associated with tension, but the cause may not be known. Pain may be associated with muscle spasm.

III. Clinical features

  A. Symptoms

    1. Dull, aching pain often accompanied by occipital pain and tightness across the scalp.

    2. Usually, middle-aged persons are affected.

    3. Headache is present for long periods.

    4. Pain is not throbbing.

    5. Usually not associated with nausea and vomiting.

    6. Headache may be associated with known periods of tension.

    7. No aura or neurologic deficit is present.

  B. Signs

    1. Usually, there are no signs:

      a. Blood pressure is normal.

      b. Results of funduscopic examination are normal; pupils are reactive.

      c. Results of the screening neurologic examination are normal.

      d. No febrile disease is present.

      e. The temporal arteries are nontender.

    2. The scalp may be sore.

    3. The muscles in the posterior neck may be tense and tender.

IV. Laboratory studies. None.

V. Differential diagnosis. Eliminate other major causes of headache.

A. Sinus headache. Pain is located over antrum, forehead, or around the eyes, most frequently in association with sinus congestion but sometimes in association with bacterial sinusitis. The overlying skin may be sensitive and the sinuses tender. Headache may begin at night and change sides with change in position.

B. Migraine. See Migraine Headache (Adult).

C. Hypertension. Hypertension may cause early morning headaches, but moderate hypertension does not usually cause severe headaches.

D. Systemic febrile disease.

E. Glaucoma. Pain is generally severe and is located around the orbits. It may be associated with nausea and vomiting. Pupils are fixed and semidilated with injected sclerae.

F. Brain tumor. Headache associated with brain tumor does not have a specific character but tends to be a more severe, deep-seated pain that may come and go and tends to worsen. It may occur at night and wake the patient; it may also occur in the early morning.

G. Cluster headache (Horton's headache). Cluster headache occurs at night, is generally localized to one orbit, and lasts approximately 1 hour. Intense pain associated with rhinorrhea, lacrimation, and flush is present. The pains tend to occur in clusters over a period of a few nights to weeks and then disappear.

VI. Treatment

A. Reassurance.

B. Analgesic—aspirin (325 mg per tablet), 2 tablets orally every 4–6 hours; or acetaminophen (325 mg per tablet), 2 tablets orally every 4–6 hours.

C. A mild tranquilizer, if stress is identifiable, may be added on physician's advice.

VII. Complications. Rare.

VIII. Consultation-referral

A. Tension headache that does not improve after initial therapy has begun.

B. All headaches not specifically diagnosed as migraine, sinus, or mild headache associated with hypertension.

C. Failure to resolve after 2 weeks of treatment.

IX. Follow-up

A. **Return visit** in 2 weeks, or sooner if necessary.

or

B. Allow patient to initiate next visit.

Vasovagal Syncope (Simple Faint): in Adults Less Than Sixty Years Old

I. **Definition.** A transient loss of consciousness and motor function due to a transient, reversible decrease in general cerebral blood flow.

II. **Etiology.** Vasovagal syncope is the result of a complex phenomenon involving, in part, vagal nerve stimulation with resultant bradycardia and venous pooling of blood in the extremities and viscera. It is often triggered by emotional factors, such as venipuncture or disturbing news. The cardiovascular phenomena are transient, lasting only a few minutes.

III. **Clinical features**

A. **Symptoms**

1. Loss of consciousness preceded by a sensation of faintness often associated with slight nausea and mild diaphoresis.

2. No headache or localizing neurologic symptoms.

3. Prompt return of consciousness, with no postictal state.

4. No history of organic heart disease, such as angina or arrhythmias.

B. **Signs**

1. Weak, thready pulse, often with bradycardia.

2. Blood pressure during actual faint less than 70 mm Hg systolic.

3. Pallor.

4. Diaphoresis.

5. Sometimes, twitching of extremities, but no definite seizure activity.

6. No bladder or bowel incontinence.

7. No postictal confusion.

8. No demonstrable neurologic deficit in post faint evaluation.

9. No murmur of aortic stenosis.

IV. Laboratory studies

    A. Hematocrit may be obtained.

    B. Obtain electrocardiogram if arrhythmias are present on clinical examination.

V. Differential diagnosis

    A. Grand mal or other seizure disorder.

    B. Localized transient cerebral ischemia, as in stroke syndromes.

    C. Syncope occurring with aortic stenosis.

    D. Syncope occurring with tachycardia or bradycardia associated with organic heart disease.

VI. Treatment

    A. Position patient so that his head is lower than his feet, or simply place him supine on the floor or ground.

    B. Record blood pressure and pulse every 5 minutes.

VII. Complications. None.

VIII. Consultation-referral

    A. Convulsion.

    B. Presence of any abnormal neurologic finding.

    C. Patient over 60 years of age.

    D. Orthostatic fall in blood pressure that persists after recovery from faint.

    E. Hematocrit reading below normal.

    F. Melena.

    G. Murmur of aortic stenosis.

    H. Arrhythmia.

    I. Failure of blood pressure and pulse to return to normal in 15 minutes.

IX. Follow-up. As needed.

Anxiety: Adult

I. Definition. State of apprehension, restlessness, nervousness, or fearfulness, which can be of long standing or relatively acute.

II. Etiology

    A. Life situations, usually associated with a family or personal crisis.

    B. Certain physical and mental illnesses.

III. Clinical features

A. Symptoms

1. Anorexia, insomnia, increased sweating, thumping in the heart, irritability, weakness and fatigue, and headaches.

2. Weight loss, nausea and vomiting, diarrhea, numbness and tingling of extremities, shortness of breath, polyuria, and amenorrhea indicate complications other than, or in addition to, simple anxiety.

B. Signs

1. Trembling of fingers, increased sweating, drawn face and tight muscles, and tachycardia.

2. Weight loss, slow speech, and flat affect indicate complications other than, or in addition to, simple anxiety.

IV. Laboratory studies. None.

V. Differential diagnosis

A. Hyperthyroidism.

B. Cancer

C. Organic brain syndrome.

D. Unexplained weight loss due to other causes.

E. Hypertension.

F. Depression.

G. Alcoholism.

H. Drug abuse.

VI. Treatment

A. Supportive therapy using staff as much as possible or frequent *short* visits to health center, or both.

B. Diazepam (Valium), 2–5 mg orally 3 or 4 times a day for a maximum of 2 weeks (controlled substance requiring physician's order).

C. Contraindications to drug therapy include:

1. First trimester of pregnancy, or if patient is near term.

2. Grief reactions (nighttime sedation is appropriate, but tranquilizers will only postpone normal grief and therefore should not be used).

3. Active liver disease.

4. Suspected drug abuse (if acute withdrawal is suspected, hospitalization is indicated).

VII. Complications

A. Drug abuse

B. Diazepam (Valium)

1. **Oversedation.** Patient should be warned that driving may be hazardous and should be urged to start drugs at time when he or she has no responsibility for driving, operating heavy machinery, and so on. If patient appears intoxicated, drug dose should be decreased.

2. **Potentiating effect.** Diazepam has a potentiating effect with other depressants, such as alcohol, tranquilizers, and narcotics if patient is undergoing treatment with such drugs, use of depressants should be avoided and consultation sought.

3. **Confusion and agitation.** These complications may occur in the elderly with depressant drug treatment. Discontinue diazepam immediately if patient becomes confused or agitated.

VIII. Consultation-referral

A. Evidence of underlying organic or other disease state, including manifestation of any of the symptoms or signs indicated as *not* consistent with simple anxiety (see **III.A** and **B.**).

B. Mental health referral is indicated if:

1. There is evidence of depressant drug abuse (e.g., concurrent use of other depressants, such as Librium, barbiturates, or alcohol). Often such a patient demands drugs but gives an unclear or vague history that is judged to be unreliable.

2. There is evidence by history that the presenting symptoms are of long standing and have not been precipitated by a real life crisis.

3. At the end of 2 weeks of treatment symptoms persist, and the patient requires continued treatment with tranquilizers.

IX. Follow-up

A. Return visit in 1 week if medication is prescribed.

B. Return visits as often as necessary, depending on severity of problem and need for continuing supportive therapy.

Tremor: Adult

I. **Definition.** Rhythmic oscillation of any part of the body, usually a distal extremity.

II. **Etiology.** Multiple causes; most commonly medication effect and diseases of the basal ganglia and cerebellum. Some elderly patients may have tremors associated with weakness or fatigue.

III. Clinical features

A. Symptoms. Usually none other than the complaint of the tremor. Patients may not notice the tremor and it may be noticed incidentally during an examination. A careful drug and alcohol history should be obtained.

B. Physical examination. A neurologic examination should be performed in all patients with tremor. The tremor should be recorded as to type (see below), and laterality. Of the many classification systems one that is widely accepted is listed below. Tremors may be of mixed types, with components of both resting and action tremor.

1. Resting tremor:
   a. Maximal at rest.
   b. May be "pill-rolling" in character.
   c. Suppressed by voluntary motion.

2. Action tremor:
   a. Maximal during activity.
   b. More rapid than resting tremor.
   c. Accentuated when patient extends arms and spreads fingers.

3. Intention tremor:
   a. Maximal during purposeful movement.
   b. Not present during beginning of activity.
   c. Increased during fine movement.

IV. Laboratory studies.
Often none indicated. Thyroid function studies indicated if suspicion of hyperthyroidism present.

V. Differential diagnosis

A. Resting tremor:
1. Parkinson's disease, other extrapyramidal disorders. Rest tremor may occasionally be seen with dementia.
2. Drug effect (phenothiazines).

B. Action tremor:
1. Benign familial tremor, which is diagnosed in the absence of other causes of action tremor.
2. Hyperthyroidism, hypoglycemia, or anxiety.

    3. Adrenergic medications, especially beta agonists such as pseu doephedrine and terbutaline.

    4. Alcohol withdrawal.

  C. Intention tremor:

    1. Cerebellar disease.

    2. Alcohol intoxication.

VI. Treatment. A tremor may be most significant as a sign of an under lying process and the general condition of the patient. Essentially never is assurance that a tremor is "part of getting old" indicated.

  A. If drug effect suspected, withdraw the offending drug after phy sician consultation. Nonprescription drugs may be withdrawn without physician consultation. Several visits may be needed to elicit alcohol history.

  B. For benign familial tremor, consult physician regarding use of pro pranolol 20–40 mg orally tid.

  C. Treatment of other tremors requires physician and sometimes spe cialty referral.

  Note: Alcohol may actually improve some types of tremor, such as benign familial tremor—such patients may be at increased risk for alcoholism.

VII. Complications. None. The severe effects of Parkinson's disease are related to the slowness of movement.

VIII. Consultation-referral. Physician should be consulted for all tremors that persist after discontinuation of nonprescription medications and ethanol.

  IX. Follow-up. As needed.

Dementia: Adult

  I. Definition. Loss of memory and other cognitive functions due to a chronic, progressive degenerative disease of the brain, leading to loss of occupational and social functioning.

  II. Etiology. More than 60 causes. Alzheimer's disease is responsible for more than 55% of dementias; it is of unknown cause and is charac terized by progressive worsening of memory and other cognitive func tions in the absence of systemic or other brain diseases that could account for the deficits. Multi-infarct dementia tends to occur in a "stepwise" progression with associated neurologic deficits. Diagnos tic tests in the workup of a patient with dementia are performed in the hope of finding a reversible cause.

III. Clinical features

A. Symptoms

1. Gradually increasing forgetfulness, especially for recent events (objects around the house, what's on the stove).

2. Decreased self-care.

3. The patient may or may not be aware of the change, or may deny any problem. The loss may have been gradual over years or relatively acute. Clear understanding of clinical course is essential to the etiologic and prognostic assessment. Often family or co-workers are the first to report a change in function.

B. Physical examination

1. A complete physical examination should be performed, but typically may reveal no abnormalities early in the course of dementia. The examination should concentrate on the causes of potentially reversible dementia, such as cerebrovascular accidents, hypothyroidism, or anemia.

2. Careful mental status examination, such as the structured "mini mental state," must be supplemented by information from family and friends.

IV. Laboratory studies

A. Complete blood count, creatinine, glucose, electrolytes, calcium, thyroid function tests, and VDRL.

B. Other studies, such as B-12 levels and CT scans, should be performed only after physician consultation.

V. Differential diagnosis

A. Potentially reversible dementias:

1. Metabolic disorders: hypothyroidism, hypercalcemia, hyponatremia.

2. Medication effect, including sedatives, cimetidine, anti-Parkinson drugs, and many others.

3. Anemia.

4. Psychiatric disorders. Depression may commonly cause a "pseudodementia."

5. A variety of neurologic diseases, including subdural hematoma, tertiary syphilis, and normal pressure hydrocephalus.

B. Nonreversible dementias:

1. Alzheimer's disease.

2. Multi-infarct dementia.

3. Dementia due to alcoholism.

Note: More than one type of dementia may coexist in a patient, and a deterioration in the functioning of a mildly demented patient should initiate consideration of a reversible cause. Any deterioration in general health may be reflected in worsening of cognitive function.

VI. Treatment

A. Treatment of the reversible dementias depends on the cause.

B. Most dementias are not curable, and treatment is supportive.

1. Personal autonomy, maximizing the patient's mental and physical capacities, should be maintained as long as is feasible.

2. Medication should be kept to a minimum.

3. Family support groups and newsletters can improve understanding.

4. Adult day care may increase socialization and provide the family with a respite.

5. A variety of home-care services may be available. The practitioner should become familiar with local agencies, including their expertise, costs, and range of services.

VII. Complications

A. Safety at home may become compromised, with difficulty cooking or driving.

B. Inadequate nutrition.

C. Family stress.

D. Late in the course of the disease, decreased mobility, falls, and incontinence may occur.

VIII. Consultation-referral. All new cases of dementia and acute deteriorations in mental status require physician consultation.

IX. Follow-up. Patients and families may need follow-up every 1–3 months; however, provider availability for questions and crisis intervention is essential in the care of the demented patient.

Disorders of the Endocrine System

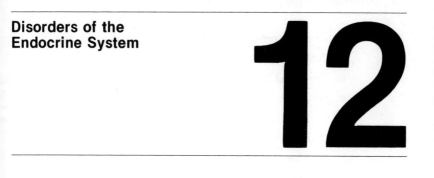

Diabetes Mellitus: Adult

I. **Definition.** Diabetes mellitus is usually an inherited disease characterized by two components:

A. **Metabolic component,** evidenced primarily by elevation of the blood glucose level.

B. **Vascular component,** leading in some patients to microvascular changes that affect the small blood vessels of the eyes, kidneys, and nerves, and macrovascular changes of accelerated atherosclerotic cardiovascular disease.

II. **Etiology**

Note: A system for classifying the various types of diabetes* has been developed by an international working group sponsored by the National Diabetes Data Group of the National Institutes of Health (NIH). This classification system has been gaining wide acceptance as a standardization of the diabetes nomenclature.

A. **Diabetes mellitus.** A broad classification covering a heterogeneous group of inherited disorders that are expressed by glucose intolerance. Within this classification are:

1. **Type I.** Insulin-dependent diabetes mellitus (IDDM), previously called juvenile, brittle, ketosis prone.

2. **Type II.** Non-insulin-dependent diabetes mellitus (NIDDM), previously called adult or maturity onset, stable, ketosis resistant. There are two subtypes:

   a. Obese.

   b. Nonobese. Some patients in this category may require insulin, but many obese Type II patients may respond to diet alone.

Diabetes, Vol. 28, December, 1979, pp. 1039–1057.

    3. Other types previously classified as secondary diabetes:

        a. Pancreatic disease.

        b. Hormonal (Cushing's syndrome).

        c. Drug- or chemical-induced:

            (1) Diuretics.

            (2) Steroids.

            (3) Phenothiazines.

            (4) Tricyclics.

        d. Insulin receptor abnormalities.

        e. Certain genetic syndromes.

B. Impaired glucose tolerance. Previously called chemical, subclinical, borderline, latent. In this condition, fasting blood sugar* is less than 140 mg per deciliter, and the blood sugar 2 hours after taking 75 gm oral glucose is elevated between normal and diabetic value (140–200 mg/dl). Another venous plasma value taken at ½, 1, or 1½ hours must also be elevated ($\geq$ 200 mg/dl).

C. Gestational diabetes

III. Clinical features

  A. Symptoms

    1. General. Although most symptoms can be attributed to glucose or vascular abnormalities, some patients may present weight loss or generalized fatigue and weakness, or both.

    2. Related to high blood glucose levels:

        a. Polyuria.

        b. Polydipsia.

        c. Polyphagia.

        d. Blurred vision to elevated glucose level in the aqueous humor of the eye.

    3. Related to vascular complications:

        a. Eyes—gradual diminution of vision.

        b. Kidneys:

            (1) Edema.

            (2) Eventually, symptoms of uremia.

*Blood sugar throughout means blood sugar level determined on venous plasma.

    c. Nervous system:

      (1) Paresthesia.

      (2) Numbness.

      (3) Weakness.

      (4) Symptoms of disturbed autonomic function (orthostatic hypotension, diarrhea, bladder difficulty, impotence).

    d. Heart—symptoms of arteriosclerotic heart disease.

    e. Peripheral vascular disease:

      (1) Cool extremities.

      (2) Claudication.

      (3) Ischemic ulcers between toes and on dorsum of the foot.

  4. Other common symptoms:

    a. Vaginal itching, usually secondary to candidal infection.

    b. Skin infections.

B. Signs

  1. Microaneurysms, hemorrhages, and exudates in ocular fundus.

  2. Evidence of advanced atherosclerosis:

    a. Coronary heart disease.

    b. Vascular insufficiency in the feet:

      (1) Poor pulses in dorsal pedis and posterior tibial arteries.

      (2) Bruits in abdomen or over femoral artery.

      (3) Ulcers between toes or on dorsum of foot.

      (4) Loss of hair on toes.

      (5) Decreased capillary filling.

      (6) Gangrene.

  3. Evidence of nervous system dysfunction:

    a. Absent knee-ankle jerks.

    b. Areas of sensory loss, particularly in the feet.

Note: Many patients with known diabetes, whether receiving treatment or not, have no symptoms or signs of diabetes or its complications.

IV. Diagnostic studies

A. Suggestive findings

1. Glucose in the urine.

2. Elevated serum glucose (this finding must be considered in relation to when the patient last ate).

3. Acetone in blood or urine (this is generally seen when diabetes is out of control or when the patient, diabetic or not, is fasting).

B. Approach to diagnosis.
A urine sugar is the best screening test for diabetes. Almost all patients who spill sugar into the urine will have an elevated blood sugar, which indicates diabetes mellitus. Not all patients with diabetes, however, spill sugar continuously. If diabetes is suspected, either a fasting blood sugar or a blood glucose drawn 2 hours after giving 75 gm of glucose orally usually is sufficient to make the diagnosis. Any of the following diagnostic criteria of the NIH working group is sufficient for diagnosis of diabetes mellitus:

1. Presence of classic symptoms; that is, weight loss, polydipsia, polyuria, ketonuria, and unequivocal elevation of plasma glucose (glucose $\geq$ 200 mg per deciliter).

2. Elevated venous plasma fasting glucose of > 140 mg per deciliter on more than one occasion.

3. Fasting blood sugar > 115 mg/dl but < 140 mg/dl. A glucose tolerance test may be used to make the diagnosis.

   a. A 75-gram glucose load is used for all patients.

   b. Blood sugar measurements every 30 minutes for 2 hours.

   c. To establish the diagnosis of diabetes mellitus, the 2-hour sample and one other must exceed 200 mg/dl.

   All abnormal glucose levels in an undiagnosed patient should lead to a physician consultation.

V. Differential diagnosis

A. Diabetes mellitus must be differentiated from other causes of hyperglycemia:

1. Chronic pancreatitis (usually secondary to alcoholism).

2. Cushing's syndrome or other normally induced hyperglycemia.

3. Drug-induced hyperglycemia.

B. Rarely, the renal threshold for glucose may be low, and urine may be positive for glucose at a normal blood level. This is known as renal glycosuria.

VI. Treatment

A. General considerations before treating hyperglycemia

1. Precipitating factors should be looked for when serum glucose rises or goes out of control in a previously stable patient. Factors to look for are:

   a. Infection.

   b. Pregnancy.

   c. Drugs, such as thiazide diuretics or corticosteroids.

2. Treatment of blood glucose should be directed at keeping the patient asymptomatic by lowering the blood sugar sufficiently to prevent polyuria and resulting dehydration and to prevent acidosis. Also, careful control of blood glucose may retard vascular complications. Therefore, close control of blood sugar is now thought to be beneficial.

3. Closer control must be maintained in those patients who are prone to develop ketosis and thus are subject to ketoacidosis. These patients include almost all juvenile diabetics.

4. Although the macrovascular disease of diabetes may not be prevented, careful skin hygiene and diligent foot care may prevent development of dangerous complications, such as gangrene and amputation.

B. Treatment of the new diabetic

1. **Evaluation**

   a. Eye examination, with testing of visual acuity and funduscopy.

   b. Examination of peripheral vascular system.

   c. Examination of nervous system.

   d. Urinalysis and determination of blood urea nitrogen and creatinine levels.

   e. Electrocardiogram and chest x-ray.

   f. Cholesterol and triglyceride levels.

2. **Diet.** Obesity is a major predisposing factor to diabetes, and all patients should attain normal weight. A diabetic reducing diet should be used until normal weight is attained and a maintenance diet developed. Restriction of calories is generally more important than restriction of carbohydrates or other specific nutrients, but fats should make up no more than 35% of calories. Diabetics should also maintain a prudent heart diet and restrict saturated fats and cholesterol to retard development of atherosclerotic disease.

Table 12-1. Comparison of urine tests by "percent"[a]

	0%		½%	1%	2%	3%	4%	5%
Clinitest two-drop method	N	T	1+	2+	3+	4+		5+
Clinitest five-drop method	N	T	1+ 2+	3+	4+			
Diastix	N	T	1+	2+	3+	4+		
Benedict's	N	1+			2+ 3+	4+		
TesTape	N	1+	2+ 3+		4+			
Clinistix	N	Light means ¼% or less; dark means ½% or more; medium means between ¼% and ½%						

[a] Percent (%) = gm/100 ml; N = normal; T = trace.

3. **Urine testing.** Urine does not correlate well with blood glucose levels. For stable diabetics, however—particularly those experienced in adjusting their own care—urine testing may be sufficient.

   a. The patient should be instructed in the proper method of collecting and testing urine and asked to keep a chart of glycosuria.

   b. Initially, urine should be tested 3 or 4 times daily.

   c. Thereafter, as the condition stabilizes, the patient may gradually decrease the frequency of testing to every other day.

   d. In follow-up, urine glucose values under 4+ will be sufficient to judge the patient's control, and therapy may be obtained on the basis of urine glucose levels alone. When levels remain at 4+, serum glucose levels are needed. Table 12-1 compares sensitivity of different urine tests to glycosuria.

4. **Self-blood-glucose monitoring.** This technique is now widely available for home care. Although more expensive than urine testing, it is becoming indispensable for managing difficult patients. Measurements are most useful when made fasting and at the times of peak activity of the insulin used.

5. **Instruction in personal hygiene,** especially foot care.

6. **Exercise:**

   a. May help patient lose weight and may decrease risk of coronary artery disease.

b. Should be encouraged in NIDDM.

c. Begin exercise at low level—consult physician.

7. Drug therapy. Beginning therapy in an obese adult with Type II NIDDM diabetes.

Note: All diabetic therapy is based on patient education. To a degree not found in any other disease, the patient manages his own therapy. Good control and maintenance require the patient to observe diet and test urine or blood at home. All manipulation of medicines is useless in the face of an uncooperative or uneducated patient.

a. If blood glucose concentration is less than 300 mg per 100 ml and the patient has no symptoms and no ketosis, institute patient education and diet.

b. If blood glucose concentration is greater than 300 mg per 100 ml, consult physician about starting oral agents or insulin. Because evidence suggests* that tolbutamide may be related to increased mortality from arteriosclerotic heart disease, oral hypoglycemic agents should be used in elderly patients who are unresponsive to diet and unable or unwilling to use insulin. Young diabetics are at greater risk for cardiovascular complications. Although the study was done against only one agent and none of the second-generation sulfonylureas, the same precautions may apply for all.

(1) Oral agents. Slowly (weekly) increase dose until symptoms are relieved or the maximum dose is reached.

(a) Tolbutamide (Orinase)—start with 500 or 1000 mg per day, given 2 or 3 times a day (maximum dose is 3000 mg).

or

(b) Chlorpropamide (Diabinese)—start with 250 mg per day, given once a day (maximum dose is 750 mg).

or

(c) Second-generation oral hypoglycemic:

(i) Glipizide (Glucotrol)—start at 5 mg once a day (maximum dose is 15 mg/day).

(ii) Glyburide (Micronase or Diabeta)—start at 2.5 mg (maximum dose is 20 mg/day).

Both drugs have 12–24 hours' duration of action

*The University Group Diabetes Program. A study of the effects of hypoglycemic agents on vascular complications in patients with adult-onset diabetes. *Diabetes* 19(Suppl.2):747–830, 1970.

and are usually started in a single dose; occasional patients may respond better to split twice-daily dosing.

(d) Side effects of oral agents include: Hypoglycemia (more common in elderly patients on chlorpropamide); gastrointestinal disturbances; and skin rashes, including photosensitivity. Also, a disulfiram type of reaction is possible if alcohol is ingested simultaneously.

(e) Because up to one-third of patients who initially respond to oral hypoglycemic agents will cease to respond in weeks or months, close follow-up is advised.

(f) Oral agents are contraindicated in patients with a history of episodes of coma or acidosis, ketosis, renal insufficiency, liver disease, cardiac or vascular disease, or who are alcoholics or are pregnant.

(2) Insulin. Of the several possible regimens for Type II diabetics, the simplest, to which many will respond, is single dose of intermediate acting insulin—NPH or lente. Alternatives are: mixed NPH and regular as a single dose, mixed NPH and regular split between A.M. and P.M., or a long-acting insulin (ultra lente), given once a day with regular insulin at bedtime. Below is a protocol for starting single-dose intermediate insulin. The initial dose—usually 15–10 units of isophane insulin suspension (NPH) or extended insulin-zinc suspension (lente) is sufficient—must be decided based on the patient's condition.

(a) Test a fasting blood glucose specimen on the morning of the first injection.

(b) Instruct patient on administration of insulin. Explain the care of needles and syringes (disposable ones are best). Outline injection sites. Observe patient drawing up insulin and self-administering it.

(c) Administer insulin. This is a good opportunity to instruct patient on insulin therapy and self-administration of insulin.

(d) Instruct patient on the relation of insulin to blood glucose level, and clarify time of peak effect of insulin. Peak effect of lente insulin and NPH insulin is 8–10 hours after injection.

(e) Inform patient of the symptoms and treatment of hypoglycemia.

Note: Hypoglycemia itself causes primarily central nervous system disturbances; the symptoms of anxiety, sweating, and tachycardia are caused by epinephrine. Thus confusion, abnormal behavior, or stupor may be the only signs of hypoglycemia.

(f) Give patient a chart for recording glycosuria and instruct to check initially at 7:00 A.M., 11:00 A.M., 4:00 P.M., and 9:00 P.M. If this is too frequent for patient cooperation, 7:00 A.M. and 4:00 P.M. will suffice.

(g) Test a blood glucose specimen at 4:00 to 5:00 P.M. to check peak effect of insulin.

(h) Schedule return visits at least once a week until diabetes is stable.

(i) Change dose for next morning on basis of 4:00 P.M. blood glucose level. Increase only in small increments (3–4 units at a time). Blood glucose should be evaluated each time insulin dose is changed.

C. Maintenance

1. See patient regularly, depending on adequacy of control and level of complications.

2. Evaluate fasting blood glucose on each visit until control is achieved, then monitor with urine testing or home blood glucose monitoring. Once the renal threshold is established, urine glucose levels below 4 + should be sufficient information in stable diabetics.

3. Continue regular home monitoring of urine sugar.

4. Provide constant reminders of the necessity for dietary control, with careful attention to weight (weight loss may mean poor control of diabetes as well as good diet.) Stress necessity of prudent heart diet.

5. Encourage exercise.

6. Take an ECG every 5 years in premenopausal females, and every year in all other patients over age 30.

7. Carry out urinalysis and determination of the creatinine concentration every year.

8. Perform careful funduscopic, peripheral vascular, and neurologic examinations every year.

VII. Complications

A. Vascular complications.

B. Elevated blood glucose level with resultant polyuria.

    C. Ketoacidosis in uncontrolled diabetes.

    D. Tendency of infections to be more difficult to control and to occur more frequently.

    E. Development of arteriosclerotic heart disease and peripheral vascular disease at an earlier age than nondiabetic persons.

VIII. Consultation-referral

    A. All new diabetics.

    B. Blood-glucose concentration greater than 400 mg per 100 ml.

    C. Refractory diabetes.

    D. To ophthalmologist after 10 years of insulin dependency or when diabetic retinopathy is found.

IX. Follow-up. See **VI.C.**

Gout and Hyperuricemia: Adult

    I. Definition. Gout is a disease that results from a variety of problems (usually an inborn error of metabolism) that lead to hyperuricemia associated with acute inflammatory arthritis or monosodium urate deposits or both that appear as either tophi or uric acid kidney stones, or both. Hyperuricemia, which may be asymptomatic, is defined as a serum level of monosodium urate greater than the generally accepted limits (7.5 mg/dl for males, and 6.6 mg/dl for females) using colorimetric methods.

    II. Etiology of hyperuricemia

        A. Gout from an inborn error of metabolism leading to overproduction of uric acid that is combined in some cases with decreased excretion. Only 10–20% of cases with clinically apparent gout give a family history of gout.

        B. Drugs, such as thiazide diuretics.

        C. Myeloproliferative diseases.

        D. Chronic renal disease.

        E. Obesity.

        F. Starvation.

    III. Clinical features. Although acute arthritis and kidney stones may appear with a normal uric acid, attacks are rare with uric acid less than 7.0 mg per deciliter and occur more frequently with increasing serum levels.

        A. Hyperuricemia. The patient is asymptomatic until arthritis or symptoms of kidney stones appear.

B. Acute gouty arthritis (first appearance or recurrent attacks):

1. **Symptoms**

   a. Painful, swollen joints.

   b. No systemic symptoms other than those from a moderately elevated temperature.

2. **Signs**

   a. Red, hot, tender joint, with inflammation extending into the surrounding tissue.

   b. Most often, involvement of only one joint, with a strong predilection for the joints of the feet, ankles, wrists, and hands. Classically, gout appears in the big toe (podagra). More than one joint may be affected, however. Temperature may be elevated.

C. Chronic gout

1. **Symptoms.** Patient is asymptomatic between attacks of acute gout.

2. **Signs**

   a. An elevated serum uric acid level (greater than 7.5 mg/dl) may be the only manifestation. With treatment, the uric acid level may fall to normal.

   b. Uric acid deposits (tophi) are found in only a small number of patients having an initial clinical attack of gout. Thereafter, with recurrence, the incidence of tophi increases. Tophi characteristically are found in and around joints, bursae, and subcutaneous tissue, especially around the olecranon bursa, the joints of the hand and foot, and the helix and anthelix of the ear.

   c. Uric acid kidney stones appear in about 20–30% of gouty patients.

IV. Laboratory studies

A. Acute gout

1. Usually, the serum uric acid level is greater than 7.0 mg per deciliter.

2. Examination of joint fluid obtained by needle aspiration reveals urate crystals.

3. White blood cell count usually is greater than 10,000 per cubic millimeter.

4. Erythrocyte sedimentation rate may be elevated.

B. Chronic gout

1. Serum uric acid level may be below normal, normal, or elevated.

2. Erythrocyte sedimentation rate is normal.

3. White blood cell count is normal.

V. Differential diagnosis. Acute gout.

A. Acute inflammatory monarthritis.

Note: In almost all new cases of acute arthritis, particularly mon-articular arthritis, the joint should be aspirated and the synovial fluid examined for bacteria and crystals.

1. Rheumatoid arthritis.

2. Pyogenic arthritis.

3. Pseudogout (chondrocalcinosis secondary to deposits of calcium pyrophosphate).

4. Reiter's disease.

5. Sarcoidosis.

B. Chronic recurrent arthritis (degenerative arthritis).

VI. Treatment

A. Description of drugs. Several drugs used in the treatment of gout have specific but different effects and must be used accordingly.

1. **Probenecid** (Benemid) blocks the reabsorption of uric acid by the proximal renal tubule. Probenecid, by causing increased ex-cretion of uric acid, lowers the serum uric acid level. This drug is not of benefit in acute gout but is used in maintenance of normal uric acid levels.

2. **Allopurinol** (Zyloprim) blocks the production of uric acid and thus decreases the serum uric acid level. This drug is used in maintenance therapy and is contraindicated in acute gout.

3. **Colchicine** has been used for many years for acute attacks of gouty arthritis. Colchicine's specific effect in terminating an acute attack of gout has diagnostic significance. It is rarely used in maintenance therapy except in patients with chronic gout who have frequent acute attacks. In this situation colchicine may reduce the frequency and severity of attacks.

4. **Indomethacin** (Indocin) and **phenylbutazone** (Butazolidin) are nonspecific anti-inflammatory drugs that frequently provide re-lief in acute gout. Other nonsteroidal anti-inflammatory drugs such as Motrin® and naprosyn have been used successfully.

B. Acute gout

1. Colchicine, 1.0–1.2 mg initially, then 0.5–0.6 mg every hour until symptoms are relieved or diarrhea, nausea, or vomiting begins. No more than 6 mg should be given for any one attack or over a 72-hour period. Pain relief usually occurs within 6–12 hours and is complete within 48–72 hours. Unfortunately GI side effects occur in more than 50% of patients.

    or

2. Indomethacin, 50 mg 3 times a day for 2–3 days, tapering to 25 mg 4 times a day for a period of 1 week (may be continued 2–3 weeks). Side effects are minimal, but gastrointestinal disturbances, headaches, rashes, and leukopenia have been reported. Other nonsteroidals may be substituted.

    or

3. Phenylbutazone, 0.4 gm initially, followed by 0.2 gm every 4 hours, to a total dose of 1 gm on days 1 and 2; then 0.1 gm 4 times a day for a maximum of 1 week. Potential hematological toxicities of phenylbutazone have been documented, but they rarely occur in short-term therapy. Other side effects include sodium and fluid retention, peptic ulceration, nausea, vomiting, and skin rashes. Because of side effects this drug is now used less frequently.

4. Rest and elevation of and cold applications to the affected joint are sometimes beneficial. Low-dose salicylates (1–2 gm per day) should be avoided.

5. Maintenance therapy with probenecid or allopurinol should not be given routinely following a first or even second attack of gout, because acute flares may be years apart. For patients with uric acid that is only mildly elevated (7.5–10 mg/dl), withhold allopurinol or probenecid until a pattern of increasing frequency is established.

C. Chronic gout

1. Known recurrent gout requires maintenance therapy with either:

    a. Probenecid, 250 mg twice a day for 1 week, then 500 mg twice a day thereafter.

       or

    b. Allopurinol, 100 mg a day for 1 week, then raise by 100 mg a day at weekly intervals until an average maintenance dose of 300 mg a day is reached.

    c. Which of these drugs to use depends upon the defect causing hyperuricemia. If a patient is excreting too much uric acid (as determined by a 24-hour urine uric acid collection), allopurinol is the drug of choice. Allopurinol is also preferred in patients with severe tophaceous gout, renal calculi, a history of renal calculi, or reduced renal function. In most other cases, however, probenecid is preferred because of the serious adverse reactions that may occur with allopurinol. For either drug, the goal of therapy is to lower the serum urate concentration to less than 7 mg per deciliter.

    d. The initial dose of either drug should be lower than maintenance dosage, because initiation of therapy may precipitate arthritis. Colchicine, 0.5–0.6 mg 2–4 times a day, may be added for several weeks during induction of therapy to prevent acute attacks.

D. Hyperuricemia. Associated with no symptom of arthritis, tophi or kidney stones.

    1. Less than 10 mg/100 ml—no therapy.

    2. Greater than 10 mg/100 ml on two successive occasions—allopurinol or probenecid (see **C.I**). Although there is a slight increased risk of renal stones or gout arthritis, many physicians may elect not to treat these patients until symptoms occur.

VII. Complications

A. Recurrent acute attacks without proper maintenance therapy can lead to chronic joint disability.

B. Untreated elevated serum uric acid level can result in:

    1. Acute gout.

    2. Renal stones with secondary infections or renal colic, or both.

    3. Tophaceous deposits in skin, joints, connective tissue.

VIII. Consultation-referral

A. New patient with acute gouty arthritis.

B. Patient known to have gouty arthritis who has frequent attacks.

C. Acute attack that persists beyond 72 hours.

IX. Follow-up

A. Chronic gout. In asymptomatic chronic gout, uric acid levels need to be checked only yearly.

B. Acute gout. The patient should be contacted or seen in 24 hours. A new patient should return in 4 weeks to discuss maintenance therapy.

Hypothyroidism—Maintenance of Diagnosed Disease: Adult

I. **Definition.** Decreased function of the thyroid gland, causing reduced production of thyroid hormone and leading to progressive slowing of all bodily functions.

II. **Etiology.** Hypothyroidism is caused by thyroid failure due to a number of mechanisms:

   A. Treatment of hyperthyroidism (radioiodine, surgery, propylthiouracil).

   B. Following thyroiditis (primarily, Hashimoto's thyroiditis).

   C. Idiopathic thyroid failure.

   D. Congenital defects in thyroid metabolism.

   E. Rarely, iodine insufficiency.

   F. Rarely, secondary hypothyroidism from pituitary or hypothalamic dysfunction.

III. **Clinical features.** The adequately treated patient should be euthyroid, without signs of hypothyroidism or hyperthyroidism:

   A. **Hypothyroidism** (secondary to inadequate treatment)

      1. **Symptoms**

         a. Decreased energy, lethargy.

         b. Cold intolerance.

         c. Constipation.

         d. Menorrhagia.

         e. Sometimes, slight weight gain late in disease.

      2. **Signs**

         a. Dry hair, which may fall out.

         b. Dry, rough skin.

         c. Hoarseness.

         d. Periorbital edema, dull expression.

         e. Slow Achilles tendon reflex (return phase).

   B. **Hyperthyroidism**

      1. **Symptoms**

         a. Nervousness.

         b. Heat intolerance.

      c. Weight loss.

      d. Increased appetite.

      e. Increased sweating.

      f. Emotional instability.

  2. Signs

      a. Sweating: moist skin.

      b. Tachycardia.

      c. Arrhythmia (primarily in older age group).

      d. Fine tremor of fingers ("cat's purr") and tongue.

      e. Lid lag.

IV. Laboratory studies (on patient being treated for hypothyroidism)

  A. Euthyroid state

Drug	T_3U	T_4
Desiccated thyroid	N	N
Synthroid (levothyroxine)	N—↑	N—↑
Cytomel (liothyronine)	↓	↓

  B. Hypothyroidism. Decreased T_3 uptake, total or free T_4, and FTI.

  C. Hyperthyroidism. Increased T_3 uptake, total or free T_4, and FTI.

  Note: Birth control pills and pregnancy increase total T_4 and decrease T_3 uptake because of increased protein substrate for binding. If both T_4 and T_3 uptake are obtained, the effects of protein substrate can be mathematically eliminated by $T_3U \times T_4$. The result of this manipulation is called the free thyroid index (FTI). The indirect FTI is generally more readily available and less expensive than a direct measure of free T_4. T_3 uptake and T_4 cannot accurately measure the level of Cytomel (synthetic T_3). Therefore these values are decreased in a patient maintained on Cytomel who is clinically euthyroid. A TSH (thyroid-stimulating hormone) is useful in diagnosis, but not necessary in patients known to have hypothyroidism.

V. Differential diagnosis. If laboratory data do not reveal any evidence of thyroid dysfunction, one must find other causes of the symptoms and clinical findings.

VI. Treatment

  A. Continue replacement therapy, adjusting according to clinical response and laboratory findings.

  B. Usual doses of thyroid replacement:

  1. Thyroid extract, 1½–2½ grains orally every day.

  2. Sodium levothyroxine (Synthroid), 0.1–0.3 mg orally every day.

  3. Sodium liothyronine (Cytomel), 25–75 μg orally in 2 divided doses a day.

VII. Complications

  A. Hypothyroidism.

  B. Hyperthyroidism.

VIII. Consultation-referral. Development of hyperthyroid signs and symptoms.

IX. Follow-up. Laboratory tests of thyroid function approximately once a year, or when patient's condition changes.

Multinodular Goiter: Adult

I. Definition. Enlargement of the thyroid in which more than one nodule is identifiable; occurs in females 10–20 times more frequently than in males.

II. Etiology. Unknown. An inborn metabolic block may be responsible. Today this disorder is very rarely secondary to iodine deficiency in the United States.

III. Clinical features

A. Symptoms

  1. Usually, patients are euthyroid, although occasionally after many years symptoms of hyperthyroidism may develop.

  2. Symptoms of tracheal compression (stridor, difficult breathing) may develop if enlargement is great.

B. Signs

  1. Visible enlargement of thyroid gland.

  2. Palpable enlarged thyroid gland with more than one nodule.

  3. Enlarged thyroid is nontender and nonpulsatile.

IV. Laboratory studies. Usually, results of thyroid studies are normal, except in the rare case of hyperthyroid goiter. Obtain serum thyroxine (T_4) and serum triiodothyronine (T_3) uptake.

V. Differential diagnosis

  A. Solitary thyroid nodule.

  B. Hashimoto's thyroiditis.

VI. Treatment

A. If the patient is euthyroid, treatment is not indicated unless the gland is cosmetically disfiguring or causing obstruction. In these cases thyroid extract, 1–2 grains daily, may be used for suppressing the pituitary production of thyroid-stimulating hormone (TSH), thus reducing the size of the thyroid gland.

B. Significant compression may require surgery.

VII. Complications

A. Hyperthyroidism.

B. Tracheal obstruction.

VIII. Consultation-referral

A. Obstructive symptoms.

B. Hyperthyroidism.

C. Solitary nodule.

D. Goiter in males, especially young males.

E. A tender thyroid gland.

IX. Follow-up

A. Every 6 months if gland is medically treated.

B. Every year if untreated.

Disorders of the Hematopoietic System

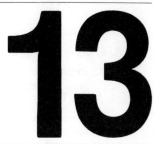

Iron Deficiency Anemia: Pediatric

I. Definition

A. Anemia in general may be defined on the basis of a lowered hematocrit reading.

Age	Hematocrit (%)
3–6 months	Less than 30
6 months–6 years	Less than 33
6–14 years	Less than 35
Over 14 years	
Female	Less than 36
Male	Less than 40

B. Iron deficiency anemia is a form of anemia resulting from an inadequate supply of iron for synthesis of hemoglobin.

II. Etiology. More than one of the following factors may be causative in an individual patient:

A. Inadequate supply of iron at birth due to:

    1. Prematurity.

    2. Fetal or perinatal blood loss without replacement.

B. Inadequate dietary iron.

C. Excessive demands for iron associated with growth:

    1. Prematurely born infant.

    2. Adolescent.

D. Blood loss without replacement:

    1. Blood loss may be obvious.

    2. The most common occult source of blood loss is the gastrointestinal tract.

III. Clinical features

A. History. One or more of the following factors may be relevant:

1. Premature birth without supplemental iron or iron-fortified milk during first year of life. Such an infant will usually be anemic by age 9 months on an average diet.

2. Iron-deficient diet. When milk not fortified with iron accounts for a large proportion of an infant's caloric intake, the overall diet will probably be poor in iron because of the low iron content of milk. Anemia from this cause is most common between 9 and 24 months of age. During the adolescent growth period, the incidence of iron deficiency anemia from an iron-deficient diet increases again, especially in females.

3. Large intake of whole cow's milk during first two years of life. This may be associated with gastrointestinal blood loss as well as a diet poor in iron.

4. Blood loss without replacement.

B. Symptoms

1. Mild iron deficiency anemia (hematocrit reading 25–33%):

   a. This condition is usually asymptomatic and discovered during routine health-maintenance screening.

   b. Results of some studies have suggested that decreased attention span may be associated with iron deficiency even before anemia develops.

2. More severe iron deficiency anemia (hematocrit reading less than 25%):

   a. Pallor.

   b. Lethargy.

   c. Irritability.

   d. Anorexia.

   e. Occasionally, poor weight gain.

C. Signs

1. Mild iron deficiency anemia—normal physical examination.

2. More severe iron deficiency anemia:

   a. Pallor.

   b. Occasional findings:

      (1) Poor weight gain.

      (2) Splenomegaly.

      (3) Systolic flow murmurs.

IV. Laboratory studies

A. Hematocrit. An abnormal value requires a repeat determination.

B. Smear of red blood cells for morphology. If anemia is more than mild, the red blood cells are hypochromic and microcytic, with some variety of size and shape.

V. Differential diagnosis

A. Anemia in general

1. Acute or chronic hemorrhage.

2. Excessive red blood cell destruction, as in hemolytic anemias such as sickle cell anemia and other hereditary anemias.

3. Decreased or impaired production of red blood cells, as in iron deficiency anemia, chronic infection, renal failure, and leukemia.

B. Iron deficiency anemia. One should try to establish why the patient is iron deficient (see **II** and **III.A**).

VI. Treatment

A. Indications for treatment without consultation. Treatment for iron deficiency anemia may be started without consultation and before results of red blood cell smear are known if *all* the following circumstances apply:

1. Hematocrit reading greater than 24% but less than normal.

2. Patient more than 10 months of age.

3. No history of a normal hematocrit or hemoglobin value in the past.

4. No history of unexplained blood loss (e.g., red blood in stools or tarry stools).

5. No history in siblings of anemia due to a cause other than iron deficiency.

6. No abnormality on physical examination not explained by an unrelated diagnosis.

B. Therapeutic measures

1. Discontinue whole cow's milk in infant under 18 months, substituting evaporated milk formula or commercial infant formula.

2. Decrease total milk intake to no more than 16 ounces a day; increase other foods, especially those with high iron content, such as iron-fortified and bran or whole cereals, dried fruit (raisins, prunes, peaches, apricots), beans (red kidney, pinto, lima, navy, soy), nuts, beef, and pork.

Table 13-1. Oral dosage of ferrous sulfate (Fer-In-Sol) (15 mg elemental iron per 0.6 ml) for treatment of iron deficiency anemia

Drug form	Body weight	Dose	Frequency
Ferrous sulfate drops (15 mg elemental iron per 0.6 ml)	8–10 kg (18–22 lb) 10–12 kg (22–26 lb)	0.6 ml* 0.9 ml*	3 times a day after meals for 2 months
or			
Ferrous sulfate syrup (6 mg elemental iron per ml)	12–16 kg (26–35 lb) 16–22 kg (35–48 lb) 22–30 kg (48–66 lb)	5.0 ml 7.5 ml 10.0 ml	3 times a day after meals for 2 months
or			
Ferrous sulfate tablets (60 mg elemental iron per tablet)	Over 30 kg (over 66 lb)	1 tablet	3 times a day after meals for 2 months

*May be given in water, fruit juice, or vegetable juice.

Table 13-2. Oral pediatric dosage of ferrous sulfate drops (Fer-In-Sol) (15 mg elemental iron per 0.6 ml) for prevention of iron deficiency anemia

Body weight	Dose*	Frequency
4–7 kg (9–15 lb)	0.3 ml	Once a day
Over 7 kg (over 15 lb)	0.6 ml	Once a day until age 18 months

*May be given in water, fruit juice, or vegetable juice.

3. Start iron therapy, 6–7 mg per kilogram of body weight (3 mg per pound) of elemental iron per day in 3 divided doses for 2 months (see Table 13-1).

C. Prevention

1. Full-term infant:

a. Breast milk.

or

b. Iron-fortified milk until age 18 months.

or

c. Medicinal iron supplement from 3–18 months of age (see Table 13-2 for dosage) unless baby consumes a solid diet with high iron content (see **VI.B.2**).

d. Intake of iron-containing foods, e.g. iron-fortified cereal.

   2. Premature infant:

   a. Iron-fortified milk until age 18 months.

   or

   b. Medicinal iron supplement from 2 to 18 months of age—ferrous sulfate drops (Fer-In-Sol) (containing 15 mg elemental iron per 0.6 ml) in a dosage of 0.6 ml once a day in water or fruit juice.

   or

   c. Breast milk and supplemental iron (see **VI.C.2.b**).

   d. Intake of iron-containing foods, e.g., iron-fortified infant cereal.

VII. Complications

   A. Progressive anemia, with increasing symptoms.

   B. Accidental ingestion of medicinal iron, especially capsules, resulting in fatal iron intoxication. Remind parents that, like all medications, it should be locked away from young children.

VIII. Consultation-referral

   A. Hematocrit reading less than 25%.

   B. Patient less than 10 months of age.

   C. History of a normal hematocrit or hemoglobin in the past.

   D. History of unexplained blood loss (e.g., red blood in stools or tarry stools).

   E. History in siblings of anemia due to a cause other than iron deficiency.

   F. Abnormality on physical examination not explained by an unrelated diagnosis.

   G. Abnormal red blood cell morphology.

   H. Failure of hematocrit to return to normal in 1 month despite iron therapy.

IX. Follow-up

   A. Clinic visit after 1 month of iron therapy:

   1. Determination of hematocrit reading (should be normal).

   2. Review of diet and further counseling as needed.

   B. Clinic visit after 2 months of iron therapy:

   1. Determination of hematocrit reading (should remain at or above 1-month level).

   2. Review of diet and further counseling as needed.

C. Clinic visit 9 months after discontinuing iron therapy:

    1. Determination of hematocrit reading (should remain normal).

    2. Review of diet and further counseling as needed.

Iron Deficiency Anemia in Menstruating Female

  I. Definition. Hematocrit reading less than 38% in menstruating females. The anemia is usually secondary to chronic iron loss and may be aggravated by intake of a diet that is low in iron as a result of food faddism or socioeconomic restrictions.

 II. Etiology. See I.

III. Clinical features

  A. Symptoms

    1. There may be none. Anemia may be discovered on routine blood examination.

    2. Fatigue, weakness, headache, dizziness, and other nonspecific generalized complaints may be present, but these symptoms rarely appear with hemoglobin levels of greater than 10 gm/dl, unless related to another problem.

    3. Heavy menstrual periods.

  B. Signs

    1. Often, there are none.

    2. Pallor of skin and conjunctiva.

    3. Fissure of lips.

    4. Brittle nails.

IV. Laboratory studies

  A. Studies required before treatment:

    1. Complete blood count, which includes:

      a. Hematocrit.

      b. White blood cell count.

      c. White blood cell differential.

      d. Red cell indices.

      e. Red cell morphology.

    2. Stool for occult blood.

B. Optional studies:

    1. Serum iron and serum iron-binding capacity.

    2. Reticulocyte count.

C. Characteristic findings in iron deficiency anemia:

    1. Hematocrit less than 38%.

    2. Normal white blood cell count.

    3. Normal white blood cell differential.

    4. Mean corpuscular volume less than 83 μ^3; mean corpuscular hemoglobin less than 27 pg (microlytic, hypochromic RBCs).

    5. Low serum iron; high serum iron-binding capacity.

V. Differential diagnosis

A. Iron deficiency anemia secondary to menstruation must be differentiated from other causes of iron loss, which frequently are due to bleeding from the gastrointestinal tract. For this reason, results of stool benzidine test must be negative.

B. Anemia secondary to ineffective production:

    1. Bone marrow depression from drugs, infections, lead poisoning.

    2. Defective hemoglobin (e.g., sickle cell).

    3. Vitamin deficiency (B_{12}, folic acid).

    4. Chronic disease.

C. Anemia from hemolysis.

VI. Treatment. Ferrous sulfate, 300 mg orally 3 times a day for 3 months.

VII. Complications. Rare.

VIII. Consultation-referral

A. Menstruating female with hematocrit reading less than 30%.

B. Menstruating female with positive stool benzidine test.

C. Failure to improve after 1 month of treatment.

D. Patients in whom serum iron or red blood cell indices, or both, do not fit iron deficiency anemia.

E. All other cases of anemia.

IX. Follow-up. Repeat hematocrit determination in 1 month.

Obstetrics and Gynecology

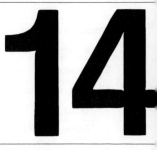

Guidelines for Managing the Obstetric Patient

I. Prenatal care. All data should be recorded on the prenatal record (Fig 14-1).

  A. The first visit

  1. Examination. The first examination should be done by the family nurse practitioner (FNP), preferably after the second missed period, unless the patient is having some trouble, such as severe nausea, vomiting, pain, or bleeding.

  a. A complete history and physical examination should be performed.

  (1) History should include questions for genetic screening:

  (a) Eastern European Jewish origin—Tay-Sachs disease

  (b) Black ancestry—Sickle cell disease.

  (c) Italian or Greek ancestry—Thalassemia.

  (d) History of spina bifida, hydrocephalus, anencephalus in family.

  (e) History of muscular dystrophy.

  (f) History of Down syndrome—how old will the patient be when the baby is born?

  (g) Bleeding problems or mental retardation in the family.

  b. The pelvic examination should include obtaining a Papanicolaou (Pap) smear and culture of the cervix for *Neisseria gonorrhoeae.*

  c. The initial laboratory work for the pregnant patient should include these studies or determinations:

  (1) Serological test for syphilis.

  (2) Blood type and Rh factor.

      (3) Antibody screening for Rh antibody.

      (4) Rubella titer.

      (5) Hematocrit.

      (6) Urinalysis and urine culture.

      (7) Tuberculin skin test.

      (8) Pap smear.

      (9) Sickle cell preparation in black patients.

     (10) Cervical culture for *N. gonorrhoeae* in high-risk populations.

2. Medications

  a. A routine prenatal vitamin with folic acid should be started at this time.

  b. Ferrous sulfate, 300 mg orally twice a day, should also be started if the hematocrit reading is below 36%.

3. Patient instruction

  a. The FNP should instruct the patient about diet and personal hygiene.

  b. The patient should be told to report to the FNP any of these conditions:

      (1) Persistent vomiting.

      (2) Continuous or severe headaches.

      (3) Persistent or recurring abdominal pain.

      (4) Vaginal bleeding.

      (5) Dimness or blurring of vision.

      (6) Chills or fever.

      (7) Loss of fluid from vagina (not vaginal discharge, but a gush of watery-type fluid or a continuous loss of this fluid).

      (8) Swelling of hands, feet, or face that becomes persistent.

      (9) Urinary symptoms, such as dysuria or hematuria.

B. The second visit

1. The second visit is made 4 weeks later.

2. Examination is done together by the obstetrician and the FNP.

3. The obstetrician should confirm the diagnosis of pregnancy, measure the pelvis, and confirm the estimated date of confinement.

Name ―――――
Race ――― Marital status (S.M.W.D. Sep.) ――― Age ――― Years married ――― Years education ――― Religion ――― Occupation ―――
Father of child
Name ―――――
Birthplace ―――
Occupation ――― Business address or employer ―――
Significant diseases ――― Height ――― Weight ――― Blood group ――― Rh ―――
Previous obstetric history
Full-term ――― Premature ――― Abortions ――― Alive ―――

No.	Year	Place of Confinement	Weeks of Gestation	Type of Delivery	Duration of Labor	Compli-cations	Apgar 1 min/ 5 min	Condition at Birth	Child Weight	Present Condition	Icterus	Rh Type	Anal-gesia	Anes-thesia
1														
2														
3														
4														
5														
6														
7														
8														
9														
10														

Eclampsia _____ Edema _____ Hyperemesis _____

Toxemia _____ Urinary tract infection _____ Rh difficulty _____

Lactation difficulty _____

Family history (tuberculosis, hypertension, heart disease, diabetes, neuropsychiatric disorders, epilepsy, allergies, multiple births, congenital anomalies)

Medical history

Blood transfusion _____ Diabetes _____ Allergy _____

Bleeding tendency _____ Hepatitis or jaundice _____ Thyroid _____

Hypertension _____ Nephritis _____ Venereal disease _____

Heart disease _____ Pyelitis, cystitis _____ Anemia _____

Phlebitis _____ Tuberculosis _____ German measles _____

Infertility _____

Operations and accidents _____

General health _____

Menstrual history

Onset at _____ years. Interval _____ days. Duration _____ days.

Irregularities _____ Dysmenorrhea _____

Coital difficulties _____

Figure 14-1. Obstetric prenatal record sheet.

Present pregnancy

Date: Last menstruation _____ Quickening _____

Expected date of

confinement: From data _____ From examination _____

Contraceptive used _____ When discontinued _____ Pregnancy planned _____

Headache _____ Vomiting _____ Indigestion _____ Constipation _____

Nausea _____ Edema _____ Vision _____ Backache _____

Leukorrhea _____ Bleeding _____ Pelvic pain _____

Height _____ Usual weight _____ Present weight _____

Remarks _____

Initial physical examination _____ Date _____

T. _____ P. _____ R. _____ B.P. _____ General nutrition _____

Oral cavity _____ Eyes _____ Optic fundi _____

Breasts _____ Nipples _____ Thyroid _____

Heart _____

Lungs _____

Kidney, liver, spleen _____

Abdominal scars _____ Height of fundus _____ Fetal heartbeat _____

Est. fetal weight _____ Presentation and position _____ Duration of pregnancy _____

Orthopedic defects _____ Varicosities _____ Edema _____

Initial pelvic examination

Outlet _____

Cervix _____

Uterus _____

Adnexa _____

Discharge _____ Rectal examination _____

Pelvic measurements

Examined by _____

T.I. _____

C.D. _____ P.S. _____ Arch. _____ C.D. _____ T.I. _____ Arch. _____

Sacrum _____ Coccyx _____ Sacrum _____ Coccyx _____

Sidewalls _____ Spines _____ SS Lig _____ SS Notch _____

X-ray pelvimetry

Date _____ Morphology _____

Trans. inlet _____ I.S. _____ T.I. _____

O.C. _____ P.S.M. _____ P.S.O. _____

Read by _____ A.P.M. _____ A.P.O. _____

Figure 14-1 (Continued)

Results of examination										
Date										
Length of gestation										
Vomiting										
Headaches										
Constipation										
Bleeding										
Upper respiratory infection										
Rash, fever										
Emotional problems										
Weight (normal)										
Weight gain/Total weight										
Edema										
Blood pressure										
Urine albumin/Urine sugar										
Hemoglobin or hematocrit										
Fetal position										
Fetal heartbeat										
Height of fundus										
Fetal weight										
Medications and immunizations										
Examiner										

Blood group _____	Rh _____	STS _____	Prenatal vitamin _____	Date _____
	Type _____	Date _____	Prenatal iron _____	Date _____
Anti-Rh titer _____	_____	_____	Parents' classes _____	
	_____	_____	Physical therapy _____	
	Type _____	Date _____		
X-rays _____	_____	_____	Analgesia preference _____	
	_____	_____	Anesthesia preference _____	
	_____	_____	Nursing preference _____	

Figure 14-1 (Continued)

C. Subsequent visits

1. **Scheduling.** Unless some special instructions are given by the obstetrician, the subsequent prenatal examinations should be done by the FNP at these intervals:

   a. Every 4 weeks until 28 weeks of gestation.

   b. Every 2 weeks from 28 to 36 weeks of gestation.

   c. Every week from 36 weeks until delivery.

2. **Routine studies**

   a. Every routine prenatal examination should include:

      (1) Questioning the patient about any present problems.

      (2) Blood pressure.

      (3) Urinalysis for protein and glucose.

      (4) Measurement of the uterine fundus.

      (5) Auscultation of the fetal heart with fetoscope or doptone, or both.

      (6) Determination of the position of the fetus, if possible.

      (7) Physical examination for edema.

      (8) Weighing the patient.

   b. Hematocrit determination should be repeated at 24 and 34 weeks in each patient, and at every visit when the patient's previous reading was below 36%.

   c. O'Sullivan screen for gestational diabetes should be done at 28–30 weeks or at initial visit if history is positive for diabetes; 50 cc of glucola orally followed by a blood glucose in one hour, glucose value of > 150 mg/dl requires a glucose tolerance test.

   d. Serum alpha feta protein (AFP) should be done at 16–20 weeks gestation.

3. **Examination.** If possible, prenatal examinations should be done by the FNP on the same day the obstetrician is to be at the clinic, but before he or she arrives, so that any problem case may be held over for review by the obstetrician.

4. **Assessment of Rh-negative patients.** At the initial prenatal screening examination, blood is drawn for blood type and Rh factor determination. All Rh-negative patients are to be handled as follows:

   a. Antibody titer is measured when the patient is discovered to be Rh negative.

b. Rh antibody titer determination is repeated in Rh-negative patients at 24, 30, and 36 weeks of gestation.

c. Patients found to have a *positive* Rh antibody titer, either initially or on repeat studies, should be referred to the obstetrician.

d. Patients who are Rh *negative*, D^U *positive*, are treated as if they were *Rh positive* (that is, there is no need for antibody titer determination or use of RhoGAM). If the newborn is Rh positive, human Rh_oD immune globulin (RhoGAM) is given immediately after delivery to all unsensitized Rh-negative women to protect them against being sensitized in future pregnancies.

5. Management of miscellaneous complaints of pregnancy

a. Constipation

(1) Advise patients that this common complaint of pregnancy may be minimized by maintaining adequate fluid intake and by promoting the softening of stools through dietary intake of fruits, juices (especially prune juice), and high-fiber foods (e.g., bran).

(2) Persistent cases may be treated with any of these stool softeners and laxatives:

(a) Dioctyl sodium sulfosuccinate (100 mg), 1 capsule twice a day as needed.

(b) Psyllium hydrophilic mucilloid (Metamucil), 1 teaspoon by mouth 2 or 3 times a day as needed.

(c) Milk of magnesia, 30 cc (2 tablespoons) at bedtime as needed.

(3) Constipation persisting for more than 10 days should be evaluated by the obstetrician.

b. Headaches

(1) Nonspecific occasional headaches may be treated with acetaminophen (325 mg tablets), 1 or 2 tablets ever 4 hours as needed.

(2) Persistent, recurrent, or migraine-like headaches should be evaluated by the physician.

c. Heartburn

(1) This complaint is seen throughout pregnancy but may be especially prominent in the last trimester. It is due to esophageal reflux through the relaxed esophogastric sphincter.

(2) Liquid antacids, 30 ml taken 30–60 minutes after meals and at bedtime as needed.

(3) Elevation of the head with pillows may reduce nighttime symptoms.

(4) Calcium carbonate (a mild antacid) is also a good source of calcium.

d. Upper respiratory infections

(1) The same diagnostic and etiologic considerations as for the nonpregnant patient (see pp. 158–160) will apply.

(2) Antibiotics should be withheld until the results of the throat culture are known.

(3) Although the use of antihistamines and decongestants is not contraindicated in pregnancy, it is prudent to restrict their use to patients in whom local agents have failed to provide relief of symptoms.

(4) Nasal sprays and nose drops are more desirable as initial therapies, since their limited absorption is less likely to expose the fetus to higher doses of medications. The following agents are acceptable for use up to 10 days: oxymetazoline HCl (Afrin) *or* xylometazoline HCl (Otrivin), nasal spray or drops, applied every 8–10 hours as needed.

e. Anemia

(1) Patients with hematocrits below 33% should have this evaluation:

(a) Repeat hematocrit. If still below 33%, proceed with studies in **(b)**.

(b) Complete blood count, sickle preparation (in black patients), serum iron, reticulocyte count, and red cell indices: If these studies show iron deficiency, begin iron therapy (325 mg ferrous sulfate 3 times a day) or encourage ingestion of previous prescription. If serum iron is normal, refer to obstetrician *and* order bilirubin (direct and indirect), urine culture, and Coombs' test.

(c) Test stool guaiac in all anemic patients.

D. Consultation-referral

1. The FNP should consult with or refer the patient to the obstetrician if any of the following are noticed:

a. No fetal heart tones are heard by 22 weeks.

b. The patient feels no movement by 22 weeks or none for 1 week at any time after this.

c. Blood pressure is above 140/90 mm Hg on two checks after bed rest.

d. Patient has albuminuria or persistent edema.

e. Patient has glycosuria.

f. There is lack of regular fetal growth.

g. Late in pregnancy the FNP questions the position of the fetus, (e.g., breech or transverse lie).

h. At any time that the FNP is in doubt about the patient's status.

i. Hematocrit reading is below 33%.

j. Symptoms of pyelonephritis.

k. Significant condylomata develop.

l. Uterus size is 2 weeks greater or smaller than expected from estimated weeks of gestation.

2. *All* prenatal patients should again be reviewed with and examined by the obstetrician at 36 weeks.

E. General instruction relative to labor and delivery. At some time, preferably between 28 and 32 weeks, but certainly before 36 weeks, the FNP should discuss with each patient when to go to the hospital.

1. Contractions

a. Primigravidas should usually wait until contractions are regular, at least 6–8 minutes apart, and lasting more than 30 seconds.

b. Multigravidas probably should wait until the contractions are regular and 10–15 minutes apart.

c. Instructions to patients, especially multigravidas, should be individualized according to the distance they must travel or history of previous rapid labor.

2. Rupture of the membranes. Patients should go directly to the hospital.

3. Any active bleeding (even without associated labor contractions). The patient should be instructed to go to the hospital. Discussion here should include differentiation of a small bloody mucous type of discharge from active bleeding. Explain to the patient that a bloody mucous discharge associated with contractions is a good sign that the contractions are true instead of false. A bloody mucous discharge by itself *without any contractions* may occur in the latter part of the pregnancy without indicating the immediate onset of labor.

4. Onset of active labor

   a. The patient should be instructed not to eat if she believes labor has started.

   b. She should be directed to report to the obstetrician at the hospital, who will then perform a vaginal examination to determine whether active labor has started. In most cases this cannot be determined on the telephone by either the FNP or the physician. The decision whether the patient will be admitted in active labor or sent home if it is false labor will be made at the time of this examination.

5. The patient should understand the various types of anesthetics available and should discuss this subject with the FNP or obstetrician. Preference for breast- or bottle-feeding should also be discussed at this time. If there are any special questions about the foregoing, they may be discussed with the obstetrician when he or she sees the patient at 36 weeks.

II. Postpartum period

A. Family planning. The FNP should discuss with the patient during pregnancy the type of birth control desired post partum:

   1. Oral contraceptives may be started upon leaving the hospital. If they are not started then, the patient should telephone the FNP within the first two weeks after returning home to obtain the pills.

   2. Intrauterine contraceptive device is no longer generally available (see Family Planning, p. 328).

   3. Postpartum tubal sterilization. Candidates for sterilization should be informed about the procedure and then evaluated by the obstetrician *before delivery.* Consent papers should be signed more than 30 days before delivery and attached to the hospital record.

   4. Diaphragm. Patient should return to the clinic at 6 weeks post partum for fitting and instructions.

B. Postpartum examinations

   1. All patients should be seen 4–6 weeks post partum for a **general physical examination, including breast and pelvic examination, plus laboratory work, including hematocrit determination and urinalysis.** These examinations should be done by the obstetrician in association *with the FNP.*

   2. A Pap smear should be done at this time if there is any question about the previous smear, or if for some reason a smear was not obtained during pregnancy.

Nausea and Vomiting During Pregnancy

I. **Definition.** Nausea or vomiting, or both, occurring during the course of pregnancy, usually during the first trimester.

II. **Etiology.** Unknown. Nausea and vomiting probably are related to the hormonal changes occurring with pregnancy, with psychologic factors playing a secondary but important role.

III. **Clinical features**

   A. **Symptoms**

      1. Nausea and vomiting, typically occurring early in the morning and then disappearing later in the day.

      2. No abdominal pain or disturbance in bowel function.

   B. **Signs**

      1. No signs of dehydration.

      2. Soft abdomen, with no tenderness. Normal bowel sounds.

IV. **Laboratory studies.** None.

V. **Differential diagnosis**

   A. Hyperemesis gravidarum.

   B. Viral gastroenteritis.

VI. **Treatment.** Advise patient on the following measures:

   A. Frequent small feedings.

   B. Antinauseant drugs: Bendectin (a combination of 10 mg-doxylamine succinate and 10 mg pyridoxine HCl per tablet), has now been taken off the market. Choice of antinauseants will depend on local preferences.

   Note: There are unpublished reports associating Bendectin with teratogenic effects, which may change its usage in the future.

VII. **Complications.** Dehydration.

VIII. **Consultation-referral**

   A. Nausea or vomiting occurring later than twentieth week of pregnancy.

   B. Dehydration.

   C. Persistence of nausea and vomiting that is annoying to patient even in the absence of dehydration.

IX. Follow-up

A. Maintain daily contact for severe nausea and vomiting.

B. Maintain weekly or less frequent contact if the problem is mild.

Candidal Vaginitis: Adult

I. Definition. An inflammatory process involving the vagina caused by a common skin fungus.

II. Etiology. *Candida albicans.* Infection often occurs in association with uncontrolled diabetes mellitus, pregnancy, antibiotic usage, and use of birth control pills.

III. Clinical features

A. Symptoms

1. Vaginal discharge.

2. Commonly, intense vulval itching or burning, or both.

3. No vaginal bleeding.

B. Signs

1. Intense vulval inflammation is commonly found.

2. Copious cheesy vaginal discharge.

3. A cheesy discharge is often present in labial folds.

4. Satellite lesions apart from the main area of inflammation may be found.

IV. Laboratory studies

A. Potassium hydroxide preparation is positive for *Candida.*

B. Wet preparation is negative for *Trichomonas.*

C. Urine should be tested for glycosuria.

D. If there is a family history of diabetes or any symptoms suggestive of diabetes are present, or both, a blood glucose specimen is drawn 2 hours after eating.

V. Differential diagnosis

A. Other causes of vaginitis.

B. Carcinoma of the vagina or cervix, or both.

VI. Treatment

A. If candidal vaginitis occurs in a patient with diabetes mellitus, the diabetes must be controlled before it is possible to control or cure the vaginitis.

B. Patient can use miconazole nitrate 2% (Monistat) *or* clotrimazole 1% (Gyne-Lotrimin, Mycelex-G) vaginal cream—1 applicatorful inserted into vagina at bedtime for 7 days or Monistat 3® Dual Pack: three vaginal suppositories (insert one suppository intravaginally a night for three nights) and cream for PRN use.

C. Cool compresses may be applied to irritated vulval lesions twice a day. Instruct patient to dry the skin thoroughly before using a compress.

VII. Complications. None.

VIII. Consultation-referral

A. Refractory cases not responding to treatment in 2 weeks.

B. Patient with coexisting uncontrolled or newly diagnosed diabetes.

IX. Follow-up. As needed.

Abnormal Papanicolaou Smear Findings in an Asymptomatic Patient: Adult

I. Definition. A report on a cytologic examination of a cervical scraping taken from an *asymptomatic* patient that is read as abnormal, with abnormalities classified as follows:

A. Inflammatory reaction (class II).

B. Suggestive of malignancy, but not highly so (class III).

C. Highly suggestive of malignancy (class IV).

D. "Diagnostic" of malignancy (class V).

II. Etiology

A. Many factors may lead to abnormal findings on Papanicolaou or Pap smears, but **inflammation secondary to infections** is probably the most common cause.

B. The possibility of a **malignancy** must always be considered.

III. Clinical features. Pap smears are most commonly done as a screening procedure, and usually no complaints are present.

IV. Purpose. Early detection of cervical carcinoma (rarely, endometrial carcinoma).

V. Frequency. See Adult Health Maintenance Flow Sheet, p. 47, for frequency of routine Papanicolaou smears for detection of cervical cancer. A Papanicolaou smear should also be done if any of the following are present:

A. Symptoms or signs suggesting gynecologic disease: Obtain Pap smears when pelvic examination is performed.

B. Sexual activity prior to age 18: Obtain Pap smears on first visit

C. History of abnormal Pap smears: Perform as indicated by physician.

D. After hysterectomy:

1. If performed for benign disease such as fibroid uterus, Pap smear should be done every 3 years.

2. If hysterectomy was performed for dysplasia or carcinoma, Pap smear should be done as indicated by physician.

VI. Equipment

A. Dacron or saline-soaked cotton swab.

B. Ayer's spatula (wood or plastic).

C. Glass slide, labeled.

D. Fixation spray.

VII. Technique

A. Use Dacron or saline-soaked cotton swab to obtain endocervical specimen from endocervical canal. Be vigorous enough to ensure adequate specimen. Spread evenly on slide.

B. Use spatula to obtain a 360-degree exocervical scraping, being sure to include the squamocolumnar junction. Spread evenly on slide.

C. One or two slides may be used, but both endocervical and exocervical specimens must be obtained.

D. Spray the slide rapidly in order to avoid drying.

VIII. Interpretation. Follow-up is predicated on the appearance of the smear

A. If no atypical cells are present, follow up on a routine basis.

B. If there are inflammatory changes (common), treat causative inflammatory condition after appropriate diagnostic workup.

C. If there is mild dysplasia,

1. Treat any infection, if present, and repeat Pap smear in 6-8 weeks (mild dysplasia reverts in 90% of patients).

2. If second smear shows mild dysplasia, refer to gynecologist for colposcopy.

D. If there is moderate or severe dysplasia, carcinoma in situ, or carcinoma, refer to gynecologist for colposcopy.

Trichomonal Vaginitis: Adult

I. **Definition.** An inflammatory process involving the vagina caused by a common flagellate parasite.

II. **Etiology.** *Trichomonas vaginalis.*

III. **Clinical features**

A. **Symptoms**

1. Vaginal discharge.

2. Vulval itching.

3. No vaginal bleeding.

B. **Signs**

1. Minimal vulval inflammation.

2. Frothy, bubbly vaginal discharge.

3. Small petechial lesions on cervix and vagina.

IV. **Laboratory studies**

A. Wet preparation is positive for *Trichomonas.*

B. Potassium hydroxide preparation is negative for *Candida.*

V. **Differential diagnosis.** Other causes of vaginitis.

VI. **Treatment**

A. **Nonpregnant patient.** Metronidazole (Flagyl), 250 mg tablets— 2-gm dose (8 tablets) orally at one time for both patient and sexual partner. Avoid alcohol for 24 hours, because a disulfiram type of reaction may occur.

B. **Pregnant patient.**

1. **Before 16 weeks of gestation,** use Trimo-San vaginal cream twice daily for 7 days for control of symptoms.

2. **After 16 weeks of gestation,** use metronidazole (see **A** for dosage).

VII. **Complications.** None.

VIII. **Consultation-referral.** Refractory cases not responding to treatment in 2 weeks.

IX. **Follow-up.** As needed.

Nonspecific or Bacterial Vaginitis: Adult

I. **Definition.** An inflammation of the vagina caused by one or more bac teria.

II. **Etiology.** Various bacteria, especially *Gardnerella vaginalis*

III. **Clinical features**

   A. **Symptoms**

   1. Minimal vulval pruritus.

   2. Vaginal discharge.

   B. **Signs.** Yellowish white vaginal discharge.

IV. **Laboratory studies**

   A. Potassium hydroxide preparation is negative for *Candida.*

   B. Hanging-drop preparation is negative for *Trichomonas* and posi tive for CLUE cells.

   C. Sniff test positive (fishy odor on addition of potassium hydroxide to vagina discharge).

   D. Culture of *Neisseria gonorrhoeae* is negative.

V. **Differential diagnosis.** Other causes of vaginitis, principally *Candida* and *Trichomonas.*

VI. **Treatment**

   A. Local measures:

   1. Povidone-iodine (Betadine) douche once, followed by triple sulfa (Sultrin) vaginal cream *or* 10% sulfisoxazole (Koro-Sulf) vaginal cream *or* Trimo-San vaginal jelly twice a day for 7 days.

   2. Vinegar douche once, followed by triple sulfa (Sultrin) or Trimo San vaginal jelly twice a day for 7 days.

   3. Triple sulfa (Sultrin) *or* 10% sulfisoxazole (Koro-Sulf) vaginal cream twice a day for 7 days.

   4. Trimo-San vaginal jelly twice a day for 7 days.

   B. Metronidazole (Flagyl), 250 mg tablets—500 mg twice a day for 7 days for resistant cases; also treat partner simultaneously.

   C. If patient cannot tolerate metronidazole use, ampicillin, 500 mg 4 times a day for 10 days; treat partner with identical dosage.

VII. **Complications.** None.

VIII. **Consultation-referral.** Refractory cases not responding to treatment in 2 weeks.

IX. **Follow-up.** As needed.

Primary Dysmenorrhea

I. **Definition.** Painful menstruation occurring in the absence of any demonstrable abnormality of the pelvic organs.

II. **Etiology.** Unknown. Psychologic factors, endocrine factors involving imbalance of estrogen and progesterone, and factors relating to prostaglandins have all been implicated.

III. **Clinical features**

   A. **Symptoms.** Cramping lower abdominal pain occurring just prior to or coincident with the onset of menstruation. May be associated with systemic symptoms, including headache, nausea, and diarrhea.

   B. **Signs.** Physical examination (including abdominal and pelvic examination) reveals no structural abnormalities. In a symptomatic patient, there may be demonstrable uterine tenderness on examination.

IV. **Laboratory studies.** None indicated.

V. **Differential diagnosis**

   A. Secondary causes of dysmenorrhea

   1. Endometriosis.

   2. Pelvic inflammatory disease.

   3. Adenomyosis.

   B. Other causes of abdominal pain that may coincidentally occur with menstruation, such as urinary tract infections and appendicitis.

VI. **Treatment**

   A. Counseling and reassurance as to the probable causes of dysmenorrhea and the absence of abnormalities of the pelvic organs.

   B. Ibuprofen, 400 mg orally 3 times a day for 5 days, beginning 2–3 days before expected onset of menses.

   or

   C. Indomethacin, 25 mg orally 3 times a day for 5 days, beginning 2–3 days before expected onset of menses.

VII. **Complications.** None.

VIII. **Consultation-referral.** Refractory cases not responding to therapy.

IX. **Follow-up.** As needed.

Bartholin's Duct Abscess and Cyst

 I. **Definition.** Soft swelling within the labia minora at the juncture of its mid and lower thirds. This abnormality, which is almost invariably the result of pyogenic infection, may present as a cystic nontender mass, but often it presents as an abscess with a tender mass, with surrounding erythema and induration.

 II. **Etiology.** Usually the result of pyogenic infection. May be caused by *Neisseria gonorrhoeae.*

III. **Clinical features**

 A. **Symptoms**

 1. Pain.

 2. Dyspareunia.

 3. Tenderness.

 B. **Signs**

 1. One or both labia are swollen.

 2. Introitis is distorted.

 3. Fluctuant swelling.

IV. **Laboratory studies**

 A. Culture of cervix for *N. gonorrhoeae.*

 B. Culture abscess material for *N. gonorrhoeae.*

 V. **Differential diagnosis**

 A. Inclusion cysts.

 B. Large sebaceous cysts.

 C. Hidradenoma.

 D. Congenital anomalies.

 E. Primary cancer or secondary malignancy metastatic to vulvovaginal area.

VI. **Treatment**

 A. Antibiotics—ampicillin, 500 mg 4 times a day for 7 days.

 B. Bed rest, local or moist heat.

 C. Codeine 30 mg with acetaminophen 325 mg (Empracet #3, Tylenol #3, Phenaphen #3), 1–2 tablets every 3–4 hours as needed (controlled substance—physician consultation required).

    D. Fluctuant abscess should be incised and drained by the nurse practitioner.

    E. When lesion is quiescent, physician should decide if the duct should be incised and marsupialized, or the diseased duct and gland should be removed.

VII. Complications. Cellulitis of surrounding tissues.

VIII. Consultation-referral. None required.

IX. Follow-up

    A. Telephone contact in 24 hours to ensure response to therapy.

    B. Examination by physician in 1–2 weeks.

Family Planning: Methods of Birth Control

Changing mores now allow people to inquire about contraception at a time when scientific developments and technologic advances provide reasonable means of birth control. Indeed, birth control pills, if taken correctly, offer complete assurance against pregnancy. Because other methods are almost as effective and many women are not willing or able to take birth control pills, other methods remain popular and necessary.

For any broad group of people, one method is predictably most appropriate—for example, birth control pills for the young woman who wants *certain* protection. An individual woman, however, may need several methods during her reproductive life. Characteristically, a young couple starts out with birth control pills until they decide to have the first child. If the effects of the pills become intolerable on resumption after delivery, the relative protection of an IUD may be sufficient. Once a family is complete and sexual habits are established, condoms, diaphragms, or vasectomy may be preferred. Any method, including coitus interruptus, may work for careful couples, but no method is effective unless used by people dedicated to its success.

In the literature the success of the various methods of contraception is expressed as both method effectiveness and use effectiveness. Method effectiveness is the idealized effectiveness if the method is used properly; use effectiveness is the actual effectiveness found in practice. Most frequently the success of birth control pills is an expression of method effectiveness, whereas the success of barrier methods often is given as use effectiveness. It is obviously unfair to compare methods using different systems. The *method* effectiveness of condoms is quite high, about 98%; however, the *use* effectiveness in studies varies from 60% to 97% depending on the skill of the group being surveyed. Clearly, methods other than oral hormones can be effective, as shown in this tabulation:*

Method	Method Effectiveness (%)	Use Effectiveness (%)
Disphragm	97–98.5	71.1–98.1
Condom	97–98.5	64.0–97.0
Combination birth control pill	99.6–99.9	90.0–99.3
IUD	97.0–99.0	94.4–99.6
Withdrawal	91.0	75.0–80.0

Discussion of the various methods of birth control follows.

I. **Coitus interruptus.** Not recommended as an effective method of contraception.

II. **Rhythm method.** Defined as avoiding intercourse 4 days before and after ovulation. This method may be used successfully by some mature couples; however, it is very unreliable and difficult to teach.

III. **Condom.** Fairly reliable method when used properly. Works best in older, mature couples. These problems can be associated with condum use:

   A. Condom may break.

   B. Condom may slide upward during intercourse or be left behind upon removal of penis.

   C. Condom must be applied before intromission.

   D. Condom must be held in place for removal of penis.

IV. **Diaphragm with spermicide**

   A. **Indications.** This method, which can be 90–95% effective when used by highly motivated couples, may be especially appropriate for breast-feeding mothers, perimenopausal women, and for women who need only occasional contraception. It may be the method of choice in women who are fearful about the systemic side effects of oral contraceptives and IUDs. The effectiveness of a diaphragm is due to the spermicidal agent (*any* spermicidal cream or jelly) used with it and to the regularity of its use.

   B. **Types.** The arching diaphragm is most frequently used, although patients who are accustomed to using a flat, non-arching diaphragm may choose to continue using that type.

---

*Tyrer, L. B., and Bradshaw, L. E. Barrier Methods. *Clinics in Obstetrics and Gynaecology* April, 1979.

C. **Fitting a diaphragm.** Diaphragms are measured according to their external diameter, ranging from 55 to 95 mm. Expertise in measuring and fitting individuals for diaphragms can be attained easily and quickly by any practitioner. Because of the risk of dislodgement at the time of orgasm, the diaphragm should be as large as can be inserted and worn without discomfort. Most patients are adept at learning how to insert and remove a diaphragm and can easily master this skill in a few minutes. Fitting of postpartum patients should be delayed until 6 weeks after delivery to allow for complete vaginal involution.

D. **Spermicidal cream or jelly.** Any spermicidal jelly or cream intended for use with a diaphragm may be used, according to personal patient preference.

V. Birth control pills

A. **Physiology.** Birth control pills suppress pituitary gonadotropins—follicle-stimulating hormone (FSH) and luteinizing hormone (LH)—which in turn suppress ovulation. Neither estrogen nor progestin effectively suppresses ovulation alone, and thus combination pills of the two hormones are required for this effect. Progestin also affects the endometrium and prevents implantation and changes the composition and consistency of cervical mucus so that sperm penetration of the mucus is decreased. Progestins alone (the "minipill") can be used for birth control but are not as effective as combinations of estrogen and progestin. The more recent triphasic combinations of estrogen and progestin appear to result in fewer unfavorable changes in serum lipids than do the standard combination pills. The new triphasic combination pills reduce the total amount of progestin dose by varying the daily dose to more closely mimic the natural hormonal flow during each cycle.

B. **Side effects.** In general, side effects are dose related, and in some cases, age related. Most problems are much less frequently seen with low-dose birth control pills.

1. Most side effects are nonspecific complaints such as bloating, nausea, edema, and cyclical weight gain and are less severe and less frequently seen with low-dose pills.

2. Thromboembolic side effects such as thrombophlebitis, CVAs, and myocardial infarction are primarily related to estrogen and are dose related; below 50 mg of estradiol no further reduction of cardiovascular side effects has been demonstrated. Progestin affects cholesterol, but clinical significance of this finding is not clear. Thromboembolic side effects greatly increase in pill takers who are over 35, smoke cigarettes, or are obese.

3. Headaches. Occur in small number of patients. In patients with migraine the effect is unpredictable.

   4. Hypertension. Occurs in a small percentage of patients. Blood pressure will usually return to normal when birth control pills are stopped.

   5. Acne may occur or be worsened in progestin-dominant BCPs.

   6. Incidence of breast and endometrial cancer is not increased.

   7. Incidence of cancer of cervix may be slightly increased.

C. Side effects from low estrogen dose

   1. Decreased menstrual flow.

   2. Amenorrhea.

   3. Breakthrough bleeding for a few months after initiation of low-dose pills.

   4. Sporadic breakthrough bleeding.

D. Contraindications

   1. Hypertension.

   2. Breast masses.

   3. Severe depression.

   4. History of phlebitis.

   5. History of embolus.

   6. Migraine headaches.

   7. Undiagnosed abnormal uterine bleeding.

   8. Impaired liver function.

   9. Myocardial infarction.

E. Relative contraindications

   1. Diabetes mellitus.

   2. Thyroid dysfunction.

   3. Leiomyomata (Fibroids).

   4. Patient aged 35 or older.

   5. Cigarette smoking.

   6. Amenorrhea.

   7. Prior to onset of regular cylces in teen-agers.

   8. Seizure disorders.

F. Types of birth control pills

1. Combination

    a. Estrogen component is either mestranol or ethynyl estradiol; these have approximately equal hormonal activity for a given weight. Because many side effects are dose related, start on the lowest dose that will prevent ovulation but will not be associated with estrogen-deficiency symptoms, usually 30–35 mg of estrogen.

    b. Progestin component—several, which have varying degrees of progestogenic properties. Theoretically, one might base the selection of a pill on physical characteristics of the patient. In practice, however, one almost always selects from a low dose of estrogen.

2. Biphasic or triphasic combination pills, which vary the progestin dose. These are as effective but have not been shown to be a significant improvement over the standard combination pill.

3. Progestin only.

4. Morning-after pill.

5. Injectable long-acting progestin.

G. Patient evaluation

1. History. Obtain history; specifically, obtain information about side effects and contraindications.

2. Physical examination. Complete physical with special attention to:

    a. Blood pressure.

    b. Breast examination.

    c. Pelvic examination.

3. Laboratory studies:

    a. Papanicolaou (Pap) smear.

    b. Blood sugar.

H. Selection of pill

1. Birth control pills offer maximum protection against pregnancy when used correctly, and are therefore an appropriate choice for anyone who absolutely does not want to get pregnant.

2. Patients should be started on the low-dose pills. Only combinations containing a low-dose estrogen (usually 30–35 mg ethynyl estradiol) are recommended.

I. Follow-up

1. Check weight and blood pressure and assess side effects after three cycles in first-time user.

2. After initial follow-up visit, annually.

3. Breast examination and Pap smear annually.

4. Return visit as necessary for problems.

J. Consultation-referral. Any persistent side effect (see **V.B**).

VI. Intrauterine devices

A. General aspects. The intrauterine device (IUD) has proved to be 95–97% effective as a contraceptive method and is especially suited to women over age 30, who may be at increased risk for oral contraceptive use. Nulliparous patients are somewhat less suitable candidates, because they are more prone to dysmenorrhea and because of the risk that salpingitis (known to be more common in IUD users) may impair future fertility. Relative contraindications include documented previous or present pelvic inflammatory disease, pregnancy, uterine fibroids, abnormal uterine bleeding, and dysmenorrhea. After approval by the consulting gynecologist, IUDs may be inserted by a nurse practitioner who has the proper training and experience. IUDs should be inserted during the menstrual period, if possible. If not, ascertain that the woman is not pregnant. Because of the medico-legal liability associated with the insertion of IUDs, it is likely that this form of birth control will soon be unavailable in the United States. Currently, the only IUD commercially available in the U.S. is the Progestasert® (ALZA).

B. Types of IUDs

1. Copper-7 and Tatum -*T*. The IUDs containing copper have been found to be more effective than those which do not contain copper (Lippes Loop). The Copper-7 and Tatum-T IUDs, however, are no longer being sold in the United States by G. D. Searle & Company (as of January 31, 1986). The decision to discontinue sales was made by the company not because of lack of confidence in the safety, efficacy, and medical utility of the product but because of escalating cost of defending product litigation. For similar reasons Ortho has discontinued distribution of Lippes Loops.

2. **Progesterone IUD (Progestasert)** releases a minute amount of progesterone into the endometrial cavity. Its significantly greater cost and limited duration of effectiveness (one year) have largely restricted its use to patients with dysmenorrhea

or menometrorrhagia, or both, in whom no other form of contraception is acceptable.

C. Side effects and complications

1. **Cramps, intermenstrual bleeding, menorrhagia.** These complaints occur more frequently among IUD users but are not indications for removal unless the patient finds them to be unacceptable in duration and degree.

2. **Pelvic infection.** Salpingitis and pelvic abscess, often unilateral, are seen with slightly increased frequency in IUD users; they are indications for removal of the device.

3. **Uterine perforation.** Difficult insertion of an IUD may lead to perforation of the device through the uterine wall. Although bleeding or unusual pain, or both, may result, often the only symptom of a perforation may be disappearance of the IUD string from its usual cervical position. Suggestion of uterine perforation requires physician consultation.

4. **Spontaneous expulsion.** Most common in the first two or three cycles but can happen at any time; may be accompanied by severe cramping and bleeding but may go undetected.

D. Removal of IUDs

1. **Indications for removal**

   a. **Partial expulsion**

      (1) The IUD is found in the vaginal vault, or the tip of the device is visualized on external or speculum examination or is palpated during bimanual examination.

      (2) This possibility must be considered when either the patient or her sexual partner complains of pain with intercourse or of feeling the device during intercourse; when the patient complains of pelvic pain or excessive bleeding; or when the patient suddenly believes the string to be longer. The cervix must be palpated very carefully, with the possibility of embedded IUD in mind.

   b. **Infection.** If the patient exhibits symptoms of uterine or pelvic infection, such as elevated white blood count (greater than 10,000), pelvic tenderness, fever, and abnormal vaginal discharge.

   c. **Pregnancy.**

   d. **Patient request.**

   e. Copper-containing IUDs may not be effective after 3 years and should be removed.

2. Procedure for removal

a. May be performed at any time in the menstrual cycle. Instruct patient that she is no longer protected against pregnancy until a new method of contraception is initiated.

b. Obtain patient history.

c. Obtain pregnancy test when indicated by patient history.

d. Perform bimanual examination to determine uterine size and position of IUD and string.

e. Insert speculum to visualize cervix; observe for IUD string.

f. Warn patient that menstrual-like cramping may occur with removal.

g. Grasp string with uterine dressing forceps and exert smooth, gentle traction on the IUD. *Do not use jerky motion.* IUD removal should be accomplished quite easily.

h. Allow patient to rest briefly after removal of device.

E. Laboratory studies

1. Complete blood count and endocervical culture if patient exhibits symptoms of endometritis or pelvic inflammatory disease.

2. Pregnancy test, if questioning pregnancy.

F. Treatment

1. Remove IUD. See **VI.D.2** for procedure.

2. Advise patient on possible complications.

VII. Post-coital birth control (morning-after pill).

In some situations postcoital birth control has become a frequently used form of birth control, particularly when unprotected intercourse occurs in circumstances in which a pregnancy would be extremely undesirable. Diethylstilbesterol (DES) in large doses was the first compound used for this purpose, and large doses of Conjugated equine estrogens (Premarin®) have also been used. Currently the treatment of choice is Ovral® (0.5 mg Norgestrel and 0.05 mg ethinyl estradiol). Two tablets stat and repeated in 12 hours, within 72 hours after intercourse. Ovral causes fewer gastrointestinal side effects and is as effective as a birth-prevention measure.

A. Consult with physician.

B. Therapy must be initiated within 72 hours of intercourse.

C. Patients should be warned that:

1. It is necessary to take all medication, despite the high incidence of nausea (with Premarin), to achieve complete effectiveness.

2. The medication is highly effective but not absolutely guaranteed to prevent pregnancy.

3. If pregnancy occurs, therapeutic abortion should be strongly considered because of possible adverse effects of the drug on the fetus.

4. Patient receiving such treatment should return in 4 weeks.

   a. Ascertain that pregnancy has been prevented.

   b. Provide contraceptive counseling.

VIII. **Therapeutic abortions.** In the United States, legal abortions are available through the second trimester. Although recent changes in federal regulations have made third-party reimbursement by Medicaid problematical and dependent on state decisions, termination of pregnancy can still be obtained through a number of sources, with tremendous regional variations. Health-care providers must acquaint themselves with the local possibilities, because diagnosis and counseling of the newly pregnant has become a major activity of some nurse practitioners. For some nurse practitioners, abortion may present a crisis of values—an understandable point of view, but one which should not conflict with a balanced presentation to patients.

Discussion of the various methods of abortion follows:

A. **Before eight weeks of gestation.** Aspiration of uterine contents with a flexible catheter is the preferred procedure. Because this removal may be done before pregnancy tests are positive, it is euphemistically called menstrual extraction. Advantages are that early aspiration may be done on an outpatient basis, with few complications.

B. **Eight to twelve weeks of gestation.** Dilation and currettage of uterine contents now has been largely replaced by curettage and vacuum procedures.

C. **Second trimester.** Several methods may be used:

   1. Intra-amniotic prostaglandin injection.

   2. Intra-amniotic injection of saline or urea.

   3. Dilation and evacuation, in selected circumstances.

   4. Rarely, direct removal of contents by vaginal or abdominal hysterotomy.

IX. **Permanent contraception**

A. **Vasectomy** (male)

   1. This procedure is 99% effective.

   2. Reanastomosis is unreliable.

   3. Psychosexual problems are occasionally reported.

    4. Of males who have a vasectomy, 50–60% will develop antibodies to sperm that can cause sterility.

B. Tubal ligation (female)

    1. Laparoscopic techniques now used have reduced hospital stay and morbidity.

    2. This procedure is 99% effective.

    3. Psychosexual problems have been reported.

Menopause

  I. Definition. Strictly speaking, menopause is the physiologic cessation of menstruation due to the normal aging of the ovary. In many women, this event occurs with few, if any, associated symptoms. In others, many associated symptoms lead them to seek medical care.

 II. Etiology. A complex and poorly understood interaction of factors involving hormonal changes (decreased estrogen, increased gonadotropin levels), vasomotor phenomena, and psychologic factors.

III. Clinical features

  A. Symptoms

    1. Vasomotor phenomena are manifested as episodes of flushing and sweating.

    2. Irritability, fatigue, insomnia, headaches, palpitation, dizziness.

    3. Dyspareunia, vaginal irritation, and pruritus.

  B. Signs. Atrophy and inflammation of the vaginal mucosa.

IV. Laboratory studies

  A. Cervical Papanicolaou smear to rule out malignancy.

  B. Potassium hydroxide and saline vaginal preparations to rule out other causes of vaginitis.

  C. Estrogen index of vaginal mucosa shows decreased maturation manifested by lack of superficial cells (large, flat mucosal cells found in inactive mucosa). Wet smear shows atrophic basal cells.

 V. Differential diagnosis

  A. Pregnancy and other causes of missed menstrual periods; other irregularities or abnormalities of menstruation; or both.

  B. Anxiety and other physiologic states occurring in the absence of menopause.

C. Alternative explanations for any of the nonspecific symptoms of menopause, such as irritability, headaches, and fatigue.

VI. Treatment

Note: The traditional use of estrogen replacement therapy for menopausal symptoms has evoked controversy in recent years because of several reports that show an association between prolonged estrogen therapy and endometrial carcinoma. This potential risk must be carefully considered and weighed against the benefits of such therapy before a decision is made to treat with estrogen replacement therapy. The prophylactic use of estrogens in asymptomatic patients is especially controversial, although proponents cite the prevention of osteoporosis as justification for its use.

A. Initial therapy

1. Conjugated estrogen, 1.25 mg by mouth each day for the first 25 days of each month. Omit estrogen for the remaining days of the month in order to avoid breast pain, possibly to avoid endometrial abnormalities due to continuous estrogen stimulation, and to allow withdrawal bleeding to occur.

   and

2. Medroxyprogesterone acetate, 10 mg by mouth each day to be taken with the last 10 estrogen tablets. This medication counteracts the unopposed estrogen effect on the endometrium and facilitates the occurrence of withdrawal bleeding.

B. Long-term maintenance therapy (consultation with physician required). If long-term maintenance estrogen replacement is deemed necessary by the consulting physician, then the following guidelines should be applied:

1. The dosage of conjugated estrogen should be reduced to the dose that will control symptoms (often, 0.625 mg or 0.3 mg will suffice). Reduction in dosage should be attempted after the first 4 weeks of therapy; however, 0.625 mg may be the lowest dose effective for preventing osteoporosis.

2. Progestin should be added each month to facilitate withdrawal bleeding (see **VI.A.2**).

3. Blood pressure must be followed closely to identify the small percentage of patients who develop hypertension on estrogen replacement therapy.

Note: Patients with previous hysterectomy for nonmalignant conditions do not require addition of a progestin to the estrogen replacement regimen, but should be given cyclic rather than continuous therapy to prevent continuous breast stimulation.

C. **Atrophic vaginitis.** Atrophic vaginitis, in the absence of other menopausal symptoms, may respond to conjugated estrogen vaginal cream (Premarin)—1 gm (¼ applicatorful) twice a day for 4 weeks. Any intercurrent vaginal infection must be treated specifically; see Candidal Vaginitis (Adult), **VI,** p. 317. Certain patients may require long-term therapy with a conjugated estrogen vaginal cream used 2 or 3 times a week, but the health-care provider should note that estrogen vaginal creams are absorbed and exert a systemic effect. Oral estrogen therapy may prove more convenient and equally effective.

VII. Contraindications and Complications

A. Contraindications

1. Hypertension.
2. Heart disease.
3. Thrombophlebitis.
4. Pulmonary embolus.
5. Large fibroids.
6. Stroke.
7. Sensitivity to estrogens.
8. Known or suspected pregnancy.
9. Undiagnosed genital bleeding.
10. Known or suspected estrogen-dependent neoplasm of the breast or reproductive tract.

All patients with a history of any of these conditions must be referred to the physician before estrogen replacement therapy is considered.

B. Complications

1. Possible carcinoma of the endometrium.
2. Breast pain.
3. Hypertension.
4. Thrombophlebitis and thromboembolia phenomena.

VII. Consultation-referral

A. All patients after first 1–2 months of therapy.
B. Any patient with a history of a contraindication.
C. Any patient who develops genital bleeding while on therapy.
D. Any patient who develops complications of therapy.

IX. Follow-up

A. Blood pressure check every 3 months for first year of replacement therapy.

B. Pap smears obtained annually while on estrogens.

C. Yearly exam for endometrial biopsy (see **VI.B.3**).

D. Frequent follow-up is needed to counsel patient and deal with psychologic and other aspects of menopausal syndrome. Goal should be to achieve asymptomatic state without use of estrogen replacement or other medications.

Pregnancy: Diagnosis and Referral

I. Definition. Although pregnancy is properly not regarded as a "disease," the process of making a diagnosis of pregnancy, which includes a pelvic examination for estimating length of gestation on the basis of uterine size, does constitute medical practice and should be covered by a protocol. This requirement is particularly applicable when the patient desires to terminate the pregnancy.

II. Clinical features (usually apparent 2 weeks after first missed period).

A. Symptoms

1. Missed menstrual period occurring in a patient whose periods are usually regular.

2. Breast engorgement.

3. Nausea or vomiting, or both, particularly in the early morning on arising.

B. Signs

1. Cervical softening (Goodell's sign).

2. Cervical and vaginal cyanosis (Chadwick's sign).

3. Softening of the uterine isthmus (Hegar's sign).

4. Enlargement of the uterus consistent with dates of pregnancy:

   a. 6 weeks—approximately two times normal size.

   b. 12 weeks—palpable on abdominal examination above symphysis pubis.

   c. 20 weeks—palpable at level of umbilicus.

   d. 36 weeks—palpable at xiphoid process.

III. Laboratory studies. Test for human chorionic gonadotropin should be positive 2 weeks after first missed period.

IV. Differential diagnosis

A. Ectopic pregnancy.

B. Menopause.

C. Other causes of amenorrhea.

D. Uterine fibromyomata.

V. Treatment

A. Enrollment in prenatal care program

or

B. Referral for therapeutic abortion after careful counseling of patient and when consistent with local laws, customs, and religious beliefs.

VI. Complications

A. See Guidelines for Managing the Obstetric Patient, **I.C.5,** for complications of pregnancy.

B. Psychologic and social complications of therapeutic abortion are frequent and often severe. Appropriate arrangements for ongoing counseling and care should be ensured.

VII. Consultation-referral

A. See Guidelines for Managing the Obstetric Patient, **I.D.,** for consultation requirements in pregnancy.

B. Therapeutic abortion. In the great majority of cases, nurse practitioners refer patients who desire a therapeutic abortion to a physician who, in some instances, may practice in a different community. The nurse practitioner should explore the alternatives and arrangements for referral of patients in advance of the need for such services. Because of the psychologic and social impact of the termination of an unwanted pregnancy, every effort should be expended to ensure proper transfer of information and continuity of care, including psychologic and social support services.

VIII. Follow-up

A. Scheduled prenatal visits; see Guidelines for Managing the Obstetric Patient, **I.C.1.,** p. 302.

or

B. Careful follow-up for patients who elect therapeutic abortion.

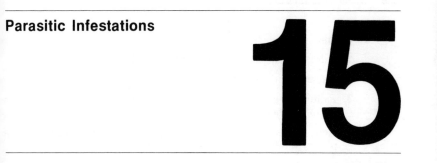

Parasitic Infestations

Ascariasis: Pediatric and Adult

I. **Definition.** Ascariasis is an infestation of the intestine by the human roundworm (*Ascaris lumbricoides*). This infestation is fairly common among young children of lower socioeconomic status in the southeastern United States.

II. **Etiology and life cycle.** Infestation begins when ascaris eggs are ingested. Children may ingest eggs by playing in or eating soil that is contaminated with eggs. Some people ingest eggs by eating unwashed, raw vegetables that were grown in contaminated soil. The soil becomes contaminated when sanitary facilities are not adequate, when infected persons (usually children) defecate directly on the ground near living quarters, or when human excrement is used for fertilizing gardens. After ingestion, the eggs hatch into larvae that migrate from the small intestine to the liver and lungs through the venous circulation. The larvae enter the alveoli of the lungs and then migrate to the trachea, where they can be coughed up or swallowed. Swallowed larvae enter the small intestine, where they mature. The adult female worms produce numerous eggs, which are passed in the stool. Individual adult worms may be passed in the stool and are easily identified on visual inspection.

III. **Clinical features**

   A. **Symptoms**

   1. Many patients are asymptomatic (likely due to infestation with only a small number of worms).

   2. Cough and fever may be present during the lung migration phase of the life cycle.

   3. Small children with large numbers of worms may have anorexia, digestive disturbances, irritability, and weight loss.

   4. Children with pica (a tendency to ingest dirt) are more likely to become infested. Pica is sometimes associated with iron deficiency anemia. Therefore, the presence of pica should prompt an evaluation for possible anemia and for ascariasis.

B. Signs

1. Adult worms may be seen in the stool.

2. Ascariasis does not cause blood loss or diarrhea.

3. Failure to gain weight may be noticed in a small child when large numbers of worms are present.

4. Acute pneumonitis (particularly if associated with eosinophilia) should suggest the possibility of ascariasis.

IV. Laboratory studies

A. None are needed if adult worms are seen.

B. Microscopic examination (by an experienced observer) of the stool of an infested person will reveal ascaris eggs.

V. Differential diagnosis

A. Pulmonary symptoms during lung migration by larvae can be confused with bacterial or viral pneumonia or asthma.

B. Other causes of failure to gain weight or of vague digestive symptoms should be ruled out.

C. Because many patients are asymptomatic, case finding can be a problem. Many cases present when an adult worm is noticed in the stool or when patients have a stool examination for eggs because of eosinophilia on peripheral blood smear.

VI. Treatment

A. Correction of poor sanitation (particularly the practice of indiscriminate defecation near houses), improvement in personal hygiene (handwashing), and care in food preparation (washing of raw foods prior to eating) are important.

B. Elimination of pica by treating iron deficiency anemia and counseling parents on proper nutrition for children.

C. Either of two drugs may be used to treat infected persons:

1. Pyrantel pamoate (Antiminth) suspension given as a single oral dose of 1 ml (50 mg) per 5 kg (10 lb) of body weight (maximum dose is 20 ml).

   or

2. Mebendazole (Vermox), 100 mg per tablet—1 tablet twice a day for 3 days (tablets may be chewed, swallowed, or crushed and mixed with food).

   Warning: Mebendazole should not be used in children under 2 years of age or in pregnant females.

VII. Complications. Rarely, intestinal obstruction results from a tangled worm mass.

VIII. Consultation-referral. Generally, not needed in routine cases.

IX. Follow-up. High-risk families with proved infection should be followed with periodic stool examinations because of the possibility of reinfection.

Pediculosis: Pediatric and Adult

I. Definition. Infestation of the skin or hair by one or both of the two species of lice capable of infesting the human host.

II. Etiology

A. *Pediculus humanis* infests the head or body.

B. *Phthirus pubis,* the crab louse, infests the genital region.

C. Both species of lice are transmitted either by close personal contact or through shared clothing, bedclothes, etc.

III. Clinical features

A. Symptoms. Intense itching.

B. Signs

1. Head (pediculosis capitis):

   a. The nits (ova) are seen as small (1-2 mm) oval objects attached to individual hair shafts.

   b. The lice themselves are difficult to find.

   c. Secondary changes in the scalp, including impetiginous changes and furuncles, may develop.

2. Body (pediculosis corporis):

   a. The lice are rarely found on the skin, but may be present in clothing.

   b. Skin lesions are characterized by changes secondary to scratching and by secondary impetiginous lesions and furuncles.

3. Genital or pubic region (phthirus pubis):

   a. As in head lice, nits may be seen on hair shafts.

   b. The lice are often difficult to find.

   c. Small black dots, which are probably excreta, may be seen.

IV. Laboratory studies. None.

V. Differential diagnosis

   A. The presence of nits or mature lice is pathognomonic.

   B. The secondary lesions, including excoriations, impetigo, and furuncles, can be of multiple origins. Their location on the scalp, pubic areas, or the skin folds may be helpful in diagnosing pediculosis.

VI. Treatment. Treatment involves proper hygiene and the use of 1% gamma benzene hexachloride (Kwell), which is available as a shampoo, cream, or lotion.

   Warning: Gamma benzene hexachloride should not be used in pregnant females or in children under 3 years of age.

   A. Hygiene. Contaminated clothing, bed linens, towels, hats, and other personal articles should be dry cleaned, washed in hot water, or dried at high heat to destroy nits and lice.

   B. Pediculosis capitis (head lice)

      1. Pyrethrins (A-200 Pyrinate, Rid), shampoo

         a. Apply to hair and scalp until hair is thoroughly wet.

         b. After 10 minutes, wash off with warm water, then shampoo hair.

         c. Remove any remaining nits with a fine-tooth comb or tweezers.

         d. Repeat application in 7–10 days.

      2. Gamma benzene hexachloride 1%, shampoo:

         a. Apply a sufficient quantity of gamma benzene hexachloride shampoo to thoroughly wet hair and adjacent hairy skin.

         b. Add small quantities of water to produce a lather and continue to shampoo for 4 minutes.

         c. Rinse thoroughly and towel briskly.

         d. Remove any remaining nits with a fine-tooth comb or tweezers.

         e. Repeat application in 7–10 days.

   C. Pediculosis corporis (body lice)

      1. Bathing plus changes of clothing and bed linens are usually sufficient for a cure.

      2. Gamma benzene hexachloride of 6–10% sulfur ointment may be used for occasional nits on body hair.

D. Phthirus pubis (pubic lice, "crabs"). Use gamma benzene hexa-chloride 1%, cream or lotion, as follows:

1. Apply liberally to hair and skin of pubic area.

2. Remove with a thorough washing after 12 hours. Rinse thoroughly and towel briskly.

3. Repeat application in 7–10 days.

4. Treat sexual contacts simultaneously.

E. Family and close contacts should be carefully examined but treated *only* if they are infested.

F. Oral antihistamines, such as diphenhydramine HCl (Benadryl), may be helpful to relieve itching (see Table 3-1, p. 96, for dosage).

VII. **Complications.** Secondary infection with impetigo, furuncles, or regional lymphadenitis, or a combination of these.

VIII. **Consultation-referral.** Questions about diagnosis.

IX. **Follow-up.** As needed.

Pinworms: Pediatric and Adult

I. **Definition.** An infestation of human pinworms (*Enterobius vermicularis*) in the intestinal tract. It is the most common parasitic infestation in the United States.

II. **Etiology and life cycle.** Infestation is initiated by the oral ingestion of pinworm eggs. Eggs from the perianal skin of infected persons (especially small children) are easily spread by hands, toys, rugs, and other objects to the hands of other persons. If hands are not washed, eggs are then transmitted from contaminated hands to the mouth. Once swallowed, the eggs hatch into larvae that mature into adult worms over the next 15–28 days as they pass through the intestinal tract. Mature female worms migrate from the anus and deposit thousands of eggs on the perineum. Pinworms can attach to the mucosa of the colon and rectum, thereby causing local irritation. The life cycle does not, however, include migration into the blood or into other tissues.

III. **Clinical features**

A. **Symptoms**

1. Patients may be asymptomatic.

2. The primary symptoms are anal pruritus and sometimes secondary skin excoriation and infection.

3. Young females may wake up crying at night with genital irritation as worms migrate into the vulval area. Such migration can also cause vulvovaginitis and dysuria.

B. Signs

1. Adult pinworms are sometimes seen on the perineum. The worms are approximately 1 cm in length and resemble white threads.

2. Perianal excoriation is sometimes present.

3. Heavy infestations (large numbers of worms in the colon and rectum) may cause perianal pain and bleeding on defecation.

IV. Diagnostic studies

A. Observation of worms by a responsible person is sufficient for diagnosis.

B. Examination for pinworm eggs will also establish the diagnosis.

1. Press a piece of clear tape (Scotch tape) directly over the anus and surrounding skin, preferably early in the morning.

2. Remove tape and place on glass slide with sticky side down.

3. Examine microscopically ($10 \times$) for characteristic eggs.

4. Do not send stool for egg examination, since eggs are primarily deposited on perianal skin.

C. Pinworms do not usually cause eosinophilia.

V. Differential diagnosis

A. Other causes of anal pruritus and excoriation (e.g., poor hygiene, localized skin infection, and anal fissure).

B. Other causes of local irritation of the female genitalia (e.g., poor hygiene, chemical irritants like bubble baths, other causes of vaginitis).

C. Other causes of dysuria (especially urinary tract infection).

VI. Treatment

A. General measures

1. Stress personal hygiene, particularly handwashing before eating and after using the toilet.

2. Pajamas and bed linens of symptomatic family members should be washed in regular laundry detergent after treatment.

B. Specific therapy (treat all symptomatic family members at the same time).

1. Pyrantel pamoate (Antiminth) suspension given as a single oral

dose of 1 ml (50 mg) per 5 kg (10 lb) of body weight (maximum single dose is 20 ml).

or

2. Mebendazole (Vermox), 100 mg per tablet—1 tablet given as a single dose (tablets may be chewed, swallowed, or crushed and mixed with food).

   Warning: Mebendazole should not be used in children under 2 years of age or in pregnant females.

VII. Complications

A. Patients may present with minor complications from localized irritation and migration (vulvovaginitis, secondary skin infection at sites of excoriation, dysuria).

B. Rarely, pinworms can cause acute appendicitis by obstructing the lumen of the appendix.

VIII. Consultation-referral. None in uncomplicated cases.

IX. Follow-up. Return visit only for recurrence.

Miscellaneous Infections

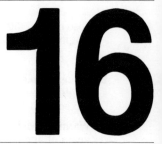

Measles: Pediatric and Adult

I. **Definition.** A highly contagious, febrile, exanthematous, viral disease associated with a high rate of serious complications.

II. **Etiology.** Measles virus.

III. **Clinical features**

    A. **Symptoms**

        1. The incubation period is 10–12 days.

        2. The catarrhal, or prodromal, period before the rash lasts 3–5 days.

            a. The patient is usually very ill, with fever up to 104°F.

            b. Coryza, cough, and conjunctivitis are prominent.

            c. Marked malaise and anorexia are present.

            d. Vomiting or diarrhea may occur.

        3. The rash usually begins on the head and neck and spreads caudally, reaching the feet on the second or third day:

            a. The fever and symptoms of the prodromal period continue after the appearance of the rash, and symptoms are most severe as the rash reaches its peak.

            b. By the second or third day of rash, the fever usually falls and symptoms begin to decrease.

            c. Fever persisting after day 4 of rash suggests the presence of complications.

    B. **Signs**

        1. Fever is present throughout the prodromal period, increasing stepwise until the height of the rash and rapidly declining on day 2 or 3 of the rash.

    2. Marked nasal discharge, conjunctivitis, and pharyngeal infection begin prodromally and continue into the rash period.

    3. Koplik's spots are pathognomonic and appear on the buccal mucosa 2 days before the rash appears.

    4. The maculopapular rash begins about the face and hairline and descends, gradually becoming confluent and eventually desquamating.

IV. Laboratory studies

    A. Paired serum samples (from the acute and convalescent periods) should be drawn and sent to state laboratories for confirmation of diagnosis.

    B. Other laboratory tests should be done on the basis of the presence of complications, after consultation.

V. Differential diagnosis

    A. Rubella.

    B. Roseola.

    C. Rocky Mountain spotted fever.

    D. Scarlet fever.

    E. Enteroviral exanthems.

    F. Drug rashes.

VI. Treatment

    A. Prevention*

        1. Live measles vaccine should be given alone or as part of combined measles-mumps-rubella vaccine as soon as possible after the age of 15 months.

        2. Adults and adolescents born after 1954, who have not had measles and who are unimmunized or who received only the killed measles vaccine, should be immunized with live measles vaccine unless there are contraindications to vaccine administration.

        3. Individuals who received measles vaccine during the first 12 months of life should be reimmunized.

    B. Therapy

        1. No specific therapy.

        2. Isolation of patient beginning with the onset of the catarrhal stage through the third day of the rash.

*See p. 4 for contraindications.

3. Immediate notification of appropriate public health authorities so that control measures may be instituted. Be certain to confirm suspected cases by obtaining serum specimens for serologic studies.

4. Investigation of immune status of family and immediate contacts, and appropriate steps to limit spread of measles.

5. Antipyretic therapy; see Chapter 5, Upper Respiratory Tract Infection (Common Cold) (Pediatric and Adult), **VI.C,** p. 159.

6. Antibiotic therapy only as indicated for specific complications.

7. Adequate fluid and nutritional intake.

8. Darkened room (this may be more comfortable, but is not necessary for conjunctivitis).

VII. Complications

A. Pneumonia

1. Pneumonia may occur at any time during the course of measles.

2. It should be treated as bacterial pneumonia, because it usually represents superimposed bacterial disease.

B. Otitis media

1. A very common complication.

2. It should be treated according to the guidelines in Chapter 5, Acute Purulent Otitis Media (Pediatric and Adult), **VI,** pp. 138–140.

C. Encephalitis

1. A very serious complication, occurring in 0.1% of cases.

2. Onset is most commonly between 2 and 6 days after the onset of the rash.

D. Tuberculosis

1. Tuberculin sensitivity is depressed during and immediately after measles.

2. Inactive tuberculosis may be activated, and children with positive tuberculin tests should be on antituberculosis therapy.

VIII. Consultation-referral

A. Consultation is indicated for all cases of suspected measles because an immediate decision needs to be made on methods to prevent the spread of the infection.

B. Patients with clinically diagnosed measles who develop signs of encephalitis should be referred immediately.

C. Consultation is indicated for patients who develop pneumonia.

D. Public health authorities should be notified immediately when suspected cases of measles are seen, and decisions should be made on steps required to limit the spread of the virus.

IX. **Follow-up.** All patients should be seen 3 or 4 days after the onset of the rash.

Infectious Mononucleosis: Pediatric and Adult

I. **Definition.** A disease primarily of children and young adults characterized mainly by fever, sore throat, enlarged lymph nodes, malaise, and lassitude.

II. **Etiology.** Epstein-Barr virus (EBV).

III. **Clinical features**

   A. Symptoms

   1. Sore throat.

   2. Malaise and lassitude.

   3. Usually, *no* nasal congestion, earache, cough, or other symptoms commonly present in respiratory infections.

   B. Signs

   1. Fever (often 101°–103°F).

   2. Inflammation of the pharynx (often exudative).

   3. Bilateral, usually nontender, enlargement of the lymph nodes. The cervical lymph nodes are almost always involved; the axillary and inguinal nodes, frequently.

   4. Often, splenomegaly.

   5. Sometimes, erythematous maculopapular rash.

   6. Periorbital edema.

   7. Sometimes, jaundice.

IV. **Laboratory studies**

   A. Throat culture is done to rule out streptococcal pharyngitis.

   B. White blood cell and differential count usually show lymphocytosis, with 10–20% atypical lymphocytes by the seventh day of illness.

   C. Heterophil antibody determination, or slide agglutination test (Monospot), is usually positive.

V. Differential diagnosis

A. Streptococcal pharyngitis.

B. Hepatitis of other origin in patients who develop jaundice.

C. Viral exanthems and other causes of skin rash.

D. Other causes of cervical lymphadenopathy and splenomegaly that have negative heterophil, such as cytomegalovirus or toxoplasma infection.

VI. Treatment

A. Acetaminophen for fever; see Table 5-5, p.151, for dosage.

B. Increased fluid intake.

C. Rest, according to degree of illness. Forced bed rest in mildly ill patient is *not* necessary.

D. Do *not* give *ampicillin* for coexisting problems in patients with infectious mononucleosis, because a rash often develops.

VII. Complications

A. Hepatitis.

B. Ruptured spleen.

C. Hemolytic anemia.

D. Aseptic meningitis.

E. Polyneuritis.

VIII. Consultation-referral

A. Splenomegaly.

B. Tender spleen.

C. Jaundice.

D. Marked tonsillar enlargement, with difficulty in swallowing.

E. Nervous system involvement.

F. Illness persisting for more than 2 weeks.

IX. Follow-up. Weekly until patient has recovered.

Mumps: Pediatric and Adult

I. Definition. Mumps is a clinical syndrome characterized by acute salivary gland enlargement, particularly of the parotid gland.

II. Etiology

A. Mumps is usually caused by mumps virus, a member of the myxo-virus family.

B. Other myxoviruses, particularly the parainfluenza viruses, can cause clinical mumps and may account for second cases of mumps and for mumps in immunized children.

III. Clinical features

A. Symptoms

1. Incubation period lasts 14–21 days, with an average of 18 days.

2. Fever may precede development of parotid swelling by 1–2 days.

3. Constitutional symptoms include headache, lethargy, anorexia, myalgia, and vomiting.

4. Parotitis produces pain anterior to the ear, which is increased by eating, local pressure, and jaw movement and is accompanied by visible swelling.

5. Symptoms related to complications (see **VII**) may *precede*, accompany, or follow parotitis.

B. Signs

1. Fever may be present.

2. Upper respiratory symptoms may accompany illness.

3. Parotid swelling is characteristic:

    a. The swelling is diffuse and difficult to demarcate.

    b. Twenty-five percent of cases have unilateral involvement.

    c. Swelling obliterates the angle of the mandible and is usually maximal near the earlobe.

    d. Stensen's duct may be inflamed.

    e. There is marked variation in the amount of parotid swelling seen with mumps.

    f. Other salivary glands may be involved.

4. Complications, particularly meningoencephalitis and orchitis (see **VII.A** and **C**), are common and should be looked for.

IV. Laboratory studies. None.

V. Differential diagnosis

A. Parotitis may be confused with the following:

1. Anterior, cervical, or preauricular lymphadenitis.

    2. Idiopathic recurrent parotitis.

    3. Parotid duct stone with secondary infection.

    4. Mikulicz's syndrome—painless bilateral enlargement of the salivary and lacrimal glands, usually with dryness of the mouth and absence of tears.

B. Meningoencephalitis may occur with or without parotid swelling and must be distinguished from other causes of meningitis.

VI. Treatment

A. Prevention

    1. Live mumps virus vaccine* should be given as combined measles-mumps-rubella vaccine after 15 months of age. Mumps vaccine is particularly recommended for persons approaching puberty and for adult males with no history of natural mumps infection or immunization.

    2. Exposed pubertal males with no history of natural mumps or immunization should be given live mumps vaccine.

    3. The value of mumps immune globulin is not established, and it is not recommended.

B. Therapy

    1. No specific treatment.

    2. Acetaminophen for fever or pain; see Table 5-5, p. 151, for dosage.

    3. Supportive care as required for specific complications.

    4. Isolation (mumps is contagious from as much as 7 days before to 9 days after parotid swelling is evident).

VII. Complications

A. Meningoencephalitis

    1. This is a very common and usually benign complication.

    2. It usually follows parotitis by 3–10 days, but may precede or occur in absence of parotitis.

    3. Hospitalization for symptomatic care may be necessary in severe cases.

B. Nerve deafness is usually unilateral, occurring after mumps.

*See p. 4 for contraindications.

C. Orchitis

1. Orchitis is usually unilateral, occurring in postpubertal males.

2. There is marked variation in the severity of symptoms. Gonadal enlargement and pain, fever, headache, nausea and vomiting, and abdominal pain all may occur.

3. Impotence does not result, and sterility is extremely rare.

D. Pancreatitis is uncommon but can be severe.

VIII. Consultation-referral. All patients with evidence of complications should be discussed with physician.

IX. Follow-up

A. Patients with complications should be checked in 24 hours, at least by telephone. Continue close follow-up until there is improvement.

B. Follow-up is not required in uncomplicated cases.

Roseola Infantum (Exanthema Subitum): Pediatric

I. Definition. Roseola infantum is an acute, benign febrile illness limited almost exclusively to children from 6 months to 3 years of age and characterized by cessation of fever as a rash appears.

II. Etiology. Unknown, but presumably a virus.

III. Clinical features

A. Symptoms

1. High fever of sudden onset lasts 1–5 days, usually 3–4 days. Fever may be sustained or intermittent.

2. There is a marked contrast between the high fever and the paucity of symptoms.

3. Symptoms, usually minimal, may include malaise, vomiting, and coryza.

4. Fever and the other minimal symptoms clear with the onset of the rash.

5. The degree of contagiousness and the incubation period are not known.

B. Signs

1. Fever occurs prior to the onset of the rash.

2. Minimal coryza, slight injection of the pharynx, and cervical and occipital adenopathy are the only clinical findings prior to the rash.

3. Rash occurs with lysis of fever:

a. Faint maculopapular rash first occurs on the trunk and neck with minimal involvement of the upper face and the extremities.

b. The rash usually clears in 24–48 hours.

IV. Laboratory studies. If a rash is not present and fever is the only abnormal finding, perform urinalysis and urine culture to rule out urinary tract infection.

V. Differential diagnosis

A. Urinary tract infection before onset of rash.

B. Rubella.

C. Other acute febrile illnesses.

VI. Treatment

A. Prevention. None.

B. Therapy

1. No specific treatment.

2. Antipyretic therapy with acetaminophen; see Table 5-5, p. 151 for dosage.

VII. Complications. Febrile seizures.

VIII. Consultation-referral

A. Seizures.

B. Fever.

1. Lasting more than 4 days.

2. Continuing after rash develops.

3. Associated with more than the minimal symptoms (see **III.A**).

IX. Follow-up. Maintain daily contact with family until diagnosis is confirmed.

Rubella: Pediatric and Adult

I. Definition. Postnatally acquired rubella is a usually mild disease associated with a 3-day rash and lymph node enlargement. Congenital infections are associated with a high incidence of congenital malformations.

II. Etiology. Rubella virus.

III. Clinical features

A. Symptoms

1. Incubation period lasts 14–21 days.

2. Transmission is by droplet spread or direct contact with infected persons or by exposure to material freshly contaminated by nasopharyngeal secretions, feces, or urine.

3. Prodromal symptoms either are absent or consist of minimal lethargy, anorexia, and upper respiratory tract symptoms.

B. Signs

1. The maculopapular rash begins about the face and neck, with rapid spread to the trunk and extremities. It usually disappears by the third day, with slight desquamation occasionally occurring.

2. Generalized lymphadenopathy is usually most pronounced in the suboccipital, postauricular, and cervical nodes.

3. Fever is usually of low grade or absent during the period of the rash.

IV. Laboratory studies

A. Paired serum samples separated by a 2-week interval should be submitted to the state laboratory for confirmation of the diagnosis if the patient has been in contact with pregnant women. A fourfold rise in the hemagglutination-inhibition titer confirms the diagnosis.

B. Pregnant women whose immunity to rubella is unknown and who have contact with a suspected case of rubella should have a rubella titer drawn immediately. A titer of greater than 1:8 indicates immunity, and the individual can be reassured that she is immune. A second blood specimen 4 weeks later should be obtained in individuals with titers of 1:8 or less. A fourfold rise in titer in a previously nonimmune individual documents infection, and the pregnant woman should be referred to a physician for a decision regarding possible termination of pregnancy.

V. Differential diagnosis

A. Measles.

B. Scarlet fever.

C. Roseola.

D. Infectious mononucleosis.

E. Enteroviral exanthems.

F. Drug rashes.

VI. Treatment

A. Prevention

1. Rubella vaccine* should be given at 15 months of age, either combined with measles or as combined measles-mumps rubella vaccine.

2. Emphasis should be placed on ensuring that all females in the child-bearing age or approaching puberty are immune. A single hemagglutination-inhibition titer equal to or greater than 1:8 establishes immunity. Nonimmune females should receive rubella vaccine and must use a medically acceptable method of contraception for 3 months following immunization.

3. The use of immune globulin is *not* recommended but may be considered for nonimmune females who have been exposed to rubella and who will not consider therapeutic abortion.

4. Officials of colleges and institutions where young adults congregate should require immunization for entry. Unless there are contraindications, unimmunized young adults, both male and female, should receive the vaccine.

B. Treatment

1. No specific treatment is available.

2. Antipyretic therapy may be used, but is rarely necessary; see Table 5-5, p.151, for dosage.

3. Contacts should be evaluated to determine if pregnant women are at risk.

4. Patient should be isolated while rash is present.

5. Cases should be reported to the appropriate public health authorities.

VII. Complications

A. Severe damage to the fetus if the infection occurs in a pregnant woman.

B. Polyarthralgia and polyarthritis can occur in adults following both natural disease and immunization.

C. Encephalitis is rare.

VIII. Consultation-referral

A. Consultation for all patients with complications.

B. Consultation for exposure of nonimmune pregnant women.

---

*See p. 4 for contraindications. In addition, pregnancy should be avoided for 3 months after receiving rubella vaccine.

IX. Follow-up

A. Follow-up is not needed in uncomplicated cases in which there is no exposure of nonimmune pregnant women.

B. Follow-up is needed to obtain convalescent serum samples from patient and exposed nonimmune pregnant women to confirm the diagnosis of rubella so that appropriate steps may be taken to terminate pregnancy, if desired.

Varicella (Chickenpox): Pediatric and Adult

I. Definition. An acute, usually benign, highly contagious disease of childhood associated with a pruritic vesicular rash.

II. Etiology. Varicella-zoster virus causes both chickenpox and herpes zoster.

III. Clinical features

A. Symptoms

1. The incubation period ranges from 10–23 days, with an average of 14–16 days.

2. A prodrome is usually absent in children; adolescents may have 1 or 2 days of prodromal fever, malaise, and anorexia.

3. Rash is characterized as follows:

    a. Lesions appear in crops, with rapid evolution (in 6–8 hours) of individual lesions from macule to papule to vesicle to crusting. Lesions in all stages are present at the same time in any given area.

    b. Lesions begin on the trunk and spread peripherally, with least involvement of the extremities.

    c. Oral mucous membranes frequently are involved with vesicles that ulcerate.

    d. Rash is usually very pruritic.

    e. New lesions usually occur for 3–5 days.

4. Onset of fever is usually at the time of the rash, and its severity is proportional to the degree of skin involvement of the rash.

5. Headache, malaise, and anorexia are usually related to the height of the fever.

B. Signs. Major physical findings are related to the rash (see **III.A.3**).

IV. Laboratory studies. None.

V. Differential diagnosis

A. Diagnosis usually is not a problem.

B. Chickenpox may be confused with the following:

1. Herpesvirus hominis infections.

2. Drug eruptions.

3. Impetigo.

4. Secondary syphilis.

5. Erythema multiforme.

6. Hand-foot-and-mouth disease (Coxsackie virus).

VI. Treatment

A. Prevention

1. No vaccine is available.

2. Immune globulin is not effective in preventing disease.

3. If exposed to varicella, patients receiving steroid or immuno-suppressive therapy, patients with immunologic disorders or malignant disease, and newborns should be referred immediately for consideration for varicella-zoster immune globulin (VZIG).

B. Therapy

1. Symptomatic care for skin:

   a. Fingernails should be kept short to minimize excoriation and scarring by scratching.

   b. Drying lotion (calamine) may be applied to lesions to decrease pruritus.

   c. Soap and water washing does not spread virus and does reduce secondary infection.

   d. Antipruritic—diphenhydramine HCL (Benadryl) or hydroxyzine HCI (Atarax, Vistaril)—may be helpful to control itching in some cases; see Tables 3-1 and 3-2 (pp. 96–97) for dosage.

2. Antipyretic-acetaminophen (Tylenol); see Table 5-5, p. 151, for dosage.

Note: Aspirin should *not* be used if varicella (chickenpox) is suspected, because there is evidence that it may be associated with the development of Reye's syndrome in patients with influenza or chickenpox.

3. Isolation. The disease is contagious from as early as 1–2 days before the rash appears until the lesions have crusted.

VII. Complications

A. Secondary bacterial infections (streptococcal or staphylococcal, or both).

B. Pneumonia. Primary viral pneumonia is extremely rare as a complication in children but relatively common in adults.

C. Encephalitis is a rare complication that has a better prognosis than most postinfectious encephalitides.

D. Severe disseminated disease may occur in newborns, patients receiving steroid or immunosuppressive therapy, or patients with immunologic deficiency or malignant disease.

E. Bleeding disorders occur very rarely.

F. Reye's syndrome.

VIII. Consultation-referral

A. All patients with conditions predisposing to severe disseminated disease (see **VII.D**) immediately upon exposure to chickenpox for consideration for varicella-zoster immune globulin (VZIG).

B. Development of pneumonia, bleeding problems, or central nervous system symptoms.

C. Severe secondary bacterial infections.

IX. Follow-up

A. In routine cases, no follow-up is required.

B. Patient should return in 48 hours if there is concern about secondary bacterial infection.

Index